RITA D ZAPATA

The Carnivore Solution

Discovering Optimal Health through Animal-Based Eating

Contents

Introduction

M eet Sarah, a remarkable individual who embarked on a transformative journey with the Carnivore Diet. Struggling for years with weight management, low energy levels, and ongoing digestive problems, Sarah's health felt like an uphill battle. Frustrated by the limitations of conventional diets, she decided to take a unique route.

With bravery and curiosity, Sarah adopted the Carnivore Diet, primarily composed of animal-based foods. What happened next was nothing short of amazing. As weeks turned into months, Sarah's body underwent a significant transformation. She started shedding excess weight, revealing a healthier and more energetic version of herself.

However, the impact of the Carnivore Diet on Sarah's health went far beyond just the numbers on a scale. Her energy levels surged dramatically, enabling her to live each day to the fullest.

A sustained sense of vigor permeated every aspect of her life, replacing the constant fatigue that had previously held her back.

The newfound mental clarity she experienced was even more remarkable. The mental fog that had clouded her thoughts for years lifted, revealing a sharper focus and improved cognitive abilities. Sarah was able to realize her full potential by investing more in her job, relationships, and hobbies.

The Carnivore Diet acted as a catalyst for Sarah's overall transformation; it was more than just a diet. Her ongoing gastrointestinal problems gradually improved, granting her newfound freedom and vitality.

Sharing her success story with those around her, Sarah became an inspiration to those seeking similar transformations. Her experience highlighted the power of personalized nutrition and the significant impact that a deliberate change in eating habits can have on overall well-being.

Sarah's journey stands as evidence of the Carnivore Diet's potential to awaken latent health and vitality. It's a reminder that anyone can rewrite their health narrative and unlock a brighter, more exciting future with willpower, an open mind, and the willingness to explore new avenues.

In a world inundated with diets advocating various restrictions and guidelines, the Carnivore Diet stands out as a primal yet intriguing approach. Join us as we delve into the science, benefits, and debates surrounding this unique dietary choice in 'Exploring the Carnivore Diet: Unleash Your Inner Predator for Optimal Health.'

The Carnivore Diet is rooted in the ancient practices of our hunter-gatherer ancestors, harkening back to a time when survival depended on the primal act of hunting and consuming animals. Our exploration delves into the origins of this diet, tracing its evolution from a contemporary option for enhancing health and well-being to a necessity for survival.

Prepare to delve into the fundamental principles of the Carnivore Diet as you flip through the pages of this book. We'll break down the nutritional components that make animal-derived foods essential for human health, examining the intricate interplay of proteins, fats, and micronutrients that form the core of this diet. This book offers more than just dietary guidance—it also addresses the challenges of adopting such a unique eating style and provides advice on adaptation, meal planning, and sustainability.

Our exploration extends beyond the dining table, encompassing science, fitness, and the environment. We scrutinize the scientific evidence that supports or challenges the Carnivore Diet's claims, and we share personal stories of individuals whose lives have been transformed by adopting a carnivorous lifestyle. By the time you reach the final pages, you'll have a comprehensive understanding of how to adopt the Carnivore Diet and incorporate its principles into a holistic approach to health.

Buckle up and get ready to dive deep into the Carnivore Diet. Each chapter will unveil new insights, dispel myths, and equip you with the knowledge you need to make informed decisions about your dietary journey. 'Exploring the Carnivore Diet' promises to be your definitive guide to primal nutrition, whether your goal is to enhance your health, try a new diet, or simply quench your curiosity.

Chapter 1: The Carnivore Diet

The Carnivore Diet is a dietary philosophy that strictly forbids the consumption of plant-based foods, including fruits, vegetables, grains, legumes, and nuts. It emphasizes the consumption of animal-based foods. It is a particularly strict type of low-carb, high-fat diet that only includes foods derived from animals, such as meat, fish, poultry, eggs, and small amounts of dairy products.

Fundamental Tenets of the Carnivore Diet

Consume Only Foods Derived From Animals: The main tenet of the Carnivore Diet is to only consume foods derived from animals. This includes fatty fish (like salmon and mackerel), organ meats (like liver and heart), white meats (like chicken and turkey), red meats (like beef, lamb, and pork), and some dairy products (like butter and specific cheeses).

Strict Prohibition of Plant-Based Foods: All plant-based foods, including fruits, vegetables, grains, legumes, and products derived from plants, are strictly prohibited from the diet. This means that no plant-based foods such as fruits, vegetables, grains, nuts, seeds, or oils are consumed.

Focus on Nutrient Density: Supporters of the Carnivore Diet frequently highlight the high nutrient density of animal foods, especially in terms of protein, vitamins (especially B vitamins), and minerals (such as iron and zinc). They contend that animal foods offer a wide variety of nutrients in forms that are easier for the body to absorb.

Elimination of Carbohydrates: The Carnivore Diet naturally excludes the majority of sources of carbohydrates because it avoids plant foods. As a result, the body consumes very few carbohydrates and enters a metabolic state known as ketosis, where it must rely on fats and protein for energy.

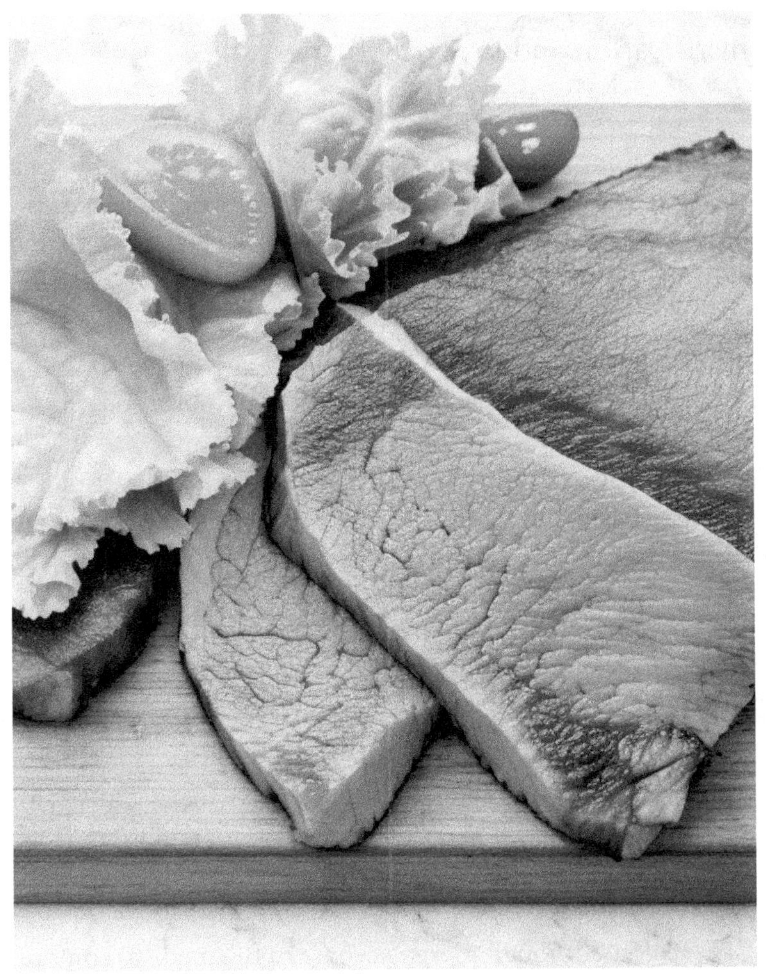

Justification and Proposed Benefits

While it's important to note that many of these claims lack strong scientific support or have limited research to back them, proponents of the Carnivore Diet suggest several potential benefits. Among the suggested advantages are:

Simplicity: The diet is easy to follow and does not require complicated meal preparation involving multiple food groups.

Weight Loss: By drastically reducing your carbohydrate intake, you may be able to lose weight by encouraging your body to use its fat reserves as energy.

Blood Sugar Regulation: The absence of carbohydrates can assist in regulating blood sugar levels and lowering insulin spikes.

Reduced Inflammation: Some people, particularly those with autoimmune diseases, report having less inflammation. However, there isn't much scientific data to back up this assertion.

Gut Health: Although there is debate in the medical community about this, proponents claim that people with digestive problems may benefit from avoiding plant fibers.

Potential Risks and Factors to Consider

The Carnivore Diet poses potential risks and concerns that need careful consideration:

Nutrient Deficiencies: Excluding plant foods may lead to deficiencies in nutrients typically obtained from fruits and vegetables, such as fiber, vitamins (like vitamin C), and minerals (such as potassium).

Constipation: The absence of dietary fiber in an all-meat diet can cause constipation, especially when transitioning suddenly.

Heart Health: While the link between saturated fat and heart disease is intricate and debated, the high intake of saturated fats from animal sources may raise concerns about cardiovascular health.

Long-Term Sustainability: Many nutrition experts worry about the impact of eliminating entire food groups on long-term health.

Lack of Research: Due to the Carnivore Diet's novelty, there's limited substantial evidence to support its claims and assess its long-term effects.

It's essential to consult a medical professional or registered dietitian before considering the Carnivore Diet, especially if you have underlying medical conditions or concerns. Despite some reported positive outcomes, this diet is a contentious option that requires cautious consideration.

Historical Background and Beginnings

The historical context and origins of the Carnivore Diet are intertwined with various historical dietary practices and cultural influences. Although the term "Carnivore Diet" might be relatively recent, the consumption of animal-based foods and the exclusion of plant-based foods have historical precedence across cultures.

Early human societies primarily consisted of hunter-gatherer communities that acquired sustenance through animal hunting and plant gathering. Depending on their environments, these societies incorporated a blend of animal and plant foods into their diets. While animal foods constituted a significant portion of their meals, it's vital to recognize that diets varied based on geographic locations and available resources.

Arctic and Inuit Diets: In regions like the Arctic, limited access to plant-based foods led Inuit populations to heavily rely on animal-based diets. Their main sources of sustenance included fatty fish, marine mammals, and other animals. The extreme Arctic climate and limited vegetation played a significant role in shaping this dietary adaptation.

Vilhjalmur Stefansson and the "No-Plants" Diet: Vilhjalmur Stefansson, an explorer who lived among the Inuit in the early 20th century, adopted their predominantly animal-based diet during his time with them. Stefansson documented his experiences and observations, contributing to the popularity of the "all-meat" or "no-plants" diet concept. It's worth noting that Stefansson's diet wasn't entirely carnivorous, as he also consumed animal organs containing essential vitamins and nutrients.

Modern Carnivore Diet Movement: In the early 21st century, the modern carnivore diet movement gained momentum primarily through social media, online platforms, and self-published books. Influential figures like Shawn Baker and Paul Saladino advocated for the benefits of exclusively consuming animal-derived foods while avoiding plant-based foods.

Proponents of this movement argue that returning to a diet resembling what they believe our prehistoric ancestors consumed could offer various health advantages, including weight loss, improved mental clarity, and relief from specific medical conditions. However, it's important to acknowledge the differing opinions among experts in science and medicine regarding the historical accuracy of these claims.

Historical Influences and Criticisms: The historical influences on the Carnivore Diet are intricate and often involve selective interpretations of traditional and ancient diets. Critics argue that these historical references are frequently oversimplified and overlook the broader context of diets and lifestyles in historical societies. Various factors, including geography, climate, and resource availability, have shaped human dietary practices, resulting in diversity and adaptability.

In Conclusion, both ancient and contemporary influences contribute to the history of the Carnivore Diet. It's crucial to approach these references with caution and a nuanced understanding of the complexity of human dietary evolution, even though some historical instances showcase primarily animal-based diets. While the modern Carnivore Diet draws inspiration from these historical examples, it has evolved into a dietary approach with its own array of claims, controversies, and considerations.

Chapter 2: Nutritional Science Behind the Carnivore Diet

To grasp the dietary implications of the Carnivore Diet and other eating patterns, understanding macronutrients—proteins, fats, and carbohydrates—and their roles in the body is essential. These macronutrients fuel various physiological processes and serve specific functions:

Proteins: Proteins consist of amino acids, the building blocks of tissues and essential components in several bodily processes. Animal-based protein sources play a crucial role in the Carnivore Diet. Proteins serve several vital roles:

Muscle Growth and Maintenance: Dietary proteins contain amino acids necessary for repairing and building muscle tissues, particularly important for individuals engaged in physical activities that demand muscle growth and repair.

Enzymes and Hormones: Proteins serve as the foundation for

many enzymes and hormones that regulate diverse biological functions such as digestion, metabolism, and fluid balance within the body.

Immune System Function: Proteins contribute to the formation of antibodies, a vital element of the immune system. Adequate protein intake supports a healthy immune response.

Fats: Dietary fats are significant energy sources and play a critical role in cellular structure and function. In a Carnivore Diet, fats are often sourced from animal products like fatty meat cuts and specific dairy items. The functions of dietary fats include:

Energy Source: Fats have a higher calorie density per gram compared to proteins or carbohydrates, making them a backup energy source when carbohydrates are scarce.

Cell Membranes: Fats are integral to cell membranes, influencing cellular structure, communication, and membrane fluidity.

Vitamin Absorption: Certain vitamins—such as A, D, E, and K—are fat-soluble, necessitating dietary fats for absorption and utilization.

Hormone Synthesis: The synthesis of hormones, including sex hormones like estrogen and testosterone, relies on the presence of fats in the body.

Carbohydrates: Carbohydrates serve as the primary energy source for the body, particularly for the brain and muscles. The Carnivore Diet, which excludes plant-based foods, virtually eliminates carbohydrate consumption. Carbohydrate functions encompass:

Glucose Production: Carbohydrates are broken down into glucose, which cells utilize as an energy source. Glucose is especially vital for meeting the energy needs of the brain.

Glycogen Storage: The liver and muscles store excess glucose as glycogen, which can be rapidly converted back into glucose when energy is required.

Dietary Fiber: While not a significant part of the carnivore diet, dietary fiber aids digestion, promotes gut health, and assists in blood sugar control. It's primarily found in plant foods.

Balancing Macronutrients: Striking a balance among macronutrients is crucial for overall health. While the Carnivore Diet emphasizes proteins and fats, it's vital to address potential nutrient gaps and ensure adequate intake of vitamins, minerals, and dietary fiber. Individual nutritional requirements vary based on factors like age, activity level, and health conditions.

Before embarking on any diet, especially one as strict as the Carnivore Diet, it's advisable to consult a healthcare professional or registered dietitian. This step ensures that your nutritional needs are met, and any risks or deficiencies are addressed appropriately.

Nutrient Content of Animal Products

The concentration of essential nutrients in a specific amount of food is known as nutrient density. Nutrient density in animal foods is a pivotal concept within the context of the Carnivore Diet, as its proponents frequently emphasize the diverse range of vital nutrients found in animal-derived products.

Animal-based foods are renowned for their high nutrient density, indicating the substantial amount of essential nutrients they offer per calorie. Among these nutrients are:

High-Quality Protein: Animal foods provide outstanding sources of high-quality protein, containing the necessary amino acids for muscle growth, maintenance, and various bodily processes.

Vitamins: Animal foods are particularly abundant in several B vitamins, including B12, B6, and riboflavin. These vitamins play crucial roles in red blood cell production, nervous system health, and energy metabolism. Additionally, certain animal products contain fat-soluble vitamins like vitamins D and A.

Minerals: Vital minerals such as iron, zinc, phosphorus, and selenium are prevalent in animal foods. These minerals are essential for maintaining healthy bones, supporting the immune system, and bolstering the body's ability to counteract free radicals.

Fats: Animal fats contain omega-3 and omega-6 fatty acids, pivotal for cellular health, inflammation control, and brain function.

Complete Nutrient Profiles: Animal foods often offer a variety of nutrients in forms that are easily absorbed and utilized by the body. For example, animal-based protein contains all the essential amino acids in optimal proportions.

Absorption and Bioavailability:

The high bioavailability of nutrients in animal foods significantly contributes to their reputation as nutrient-dense options. Bioavailability refers to the amount of nutrients in food that the body absorbs and uses. Owing to their structural similarity to human tissues, nutrients from animal sources tend to be highly bioavailable and more readily absorbed compared to certain plant-based nutrients.

Contrasting Foods from Plants and Animals

While plant foods also deliver vital nutrients, vitamins, minerals, and dietary fiber, animal foods are known for their nutrient density. The distinction lies in bioavailability and nutrient profiles. For instance, some plant foods might contain vitamins and minerals, but they could also include substances that hinder the absorption of these nutrients or necessitate specific conditions for optimal utilization.

Considering Various Factors:

A balanced diet encompasses a variety of nutrient sources, even as nutrient density remains a critical consideration. A diet exclusively composed of animal products, like the Carnivore Diet, may offer nutrient density benefits but could also carry the risk of nutrient deficiencies. It's imperative to ensure that the diet provides all the necessary vitamins, minerals, and nutrients required to sustain overall health and well-being.

Before making significant dietary changes, especially if contemplating a highly restrictive diet like the Carnivore Diet, it's advisable to consult a healthcare provider or registered dietitian. This step ensures a tailored understanding of your nutritional needs, addresses potential deficiencies, and devises a balanced plan aligned with your health objectives.

Advantages and Disadvantages of an All-Meat Diet

An all-meat diet, such as the Carnivore Diet, exclusively relies on animal-derived foods while excluding all plant-based options. Advocates of this diet present various potential advantages, but it's essential to carefully assess both the purported benefits and potential drawbacks in light of available scientific evidence and expert opinions.

Possible Advantages:

simplicity: The all-meat diet is easy to follow because it does not require complicated meal planning involving different food groups.

Loss of weight: Cutting out carbohydrates from the diet can cause ketosis, a metabolic state in which the body uses fat as fuel. Particularly in the short term, this may lead to weight loss.

blood sugar regulation: People with type 2 diabetes or insulin resistance may find that a low-carb diet, such as the all-meat diet, helps to stabilize blood sugar levels and reduces insulin spikes.

satiety: Foods high in protein and fat can make you feel full and lessen your cravings, which may help you control your appetite.

digestive problems: Some people who have particular digestive disorders, like irritable bowel syndrome (IBS), report symptom relief on an all-meat diet because there are no plant compounds present that could cause those symptoms.

Autoimmune disorders: A small percentage of people with autoimmune disorders may experience symptom relief as a result of a possible decrease in certain plant-based compounds that could provoke immune reactions.

Possible Disadvantages:

Deficiencies in vitamins, minerals, and dietary fiber—all of which are commonly found in fruits, vegetables, and grains—could result from avoiding plant foods. For instance, dietary fiber and vitamin C, both of which are found in vegetables and fruits, may be deficient.

digestive discomfort can result from a sudden switch to an all-meat diet because the lack of dietary fiber can cause constipation or alter the composition of the gut bacteria.

Concerns about cardiovascular health may arise from a diet high in animal-based saturated fats, especially in people with certain risk factors.

Long-term viability: There is disagreement regarding the viability of an all-meat diet. Due to social difficulties and a lack of food variety, the restrictive nature of the diet may eventually affect adherence.

Lack of scientific support: The long-term effects of an all-meat diet have received little attention from researchers. The majority of dietary recommendations stress the value of a varied, well-balanced diet.

Concerns about animal welfare and environmental sustainability arise from relying solely on animal products because of the greater environmental impact associated with meat production.

Potential health risks: An all-meat diet's extreme nature raises questions about possible unidentified health risks, particularly when adhered to for extended periods without medical supervision.

It is crucial to speak with a medical professional or registered dietitian before considering an all-meat diet. Depending on your goals, nutritional requirements, and current state of health, they can offer you individualized advice. While some people may claim that these diets are beneficial, the potential risks and paucity of long-term research call for careful thought and well-informed decision-making.

Chapter 3: Types of Foods Allowed on the Carnivore Diet

The Carnivore Diet relies heavily on sources of animal protein for essential nutrients like protein, vitamins, and minerals. The three main sources of animal protein are red meat, poultry, and fish, which are explained below.

1. Red Meat: Myoglobin, a protein that carries oxygen, is a component of red meat, which is the term for the muscle tissue of mammals. Red meat is frequently sourced from beef, lamb, and pork. Red meat is prized for its high protein and nutrient density.

Food Composition of Red Meat

Red meat is a great source of high-quality protein and contains all the essential amino acids that the body requires for a variety of processes, including the upkeep and expansion of muscles.

Vitamins: Red meat is a good source of B vitamins, including B12, which is necessary for the production of red blood cells and nerve function. Niacin, riboflavin, and vitamin B6 are among the additional B vitamins that are present.

Minerals: Minerals like iron, zinc, and selenium are abundant in red meat. Zinc supports immune system health and wound healing while iron is crucial for oxygen transport in the blood.

Saturated and unsaturated fats can both be found in red meat in varying amounts, depending on the cut.

2. Poultry: Domesticated birds raised for meat, like chicken and turkey, are considered poultry. Because of its lean protein content and adaptability in the kitchen, poultry is frequently preferred.

Food Composition of Poultry

Lean Protein: Poultry is a popular option for people looking to reduce their intake of saturated fat while still getting the protein they need.

B vitamins: Poultry is a good source of B vitamins like niacin, vitamin B6, and B12. This is similar to red meat.

Minerals: Phosphorus, which is crucial for bone health, and selenium, an antioxidant, are minerals found in poultry.

Low in Saturated Fat: When compared to red meat, skinless poultry is especially low in saturated fat.

3. Fish: Rich in protein, omega-3 fatty acids, and other nutrients, fish is a great source of food. Particularly prized for its omega-3 content is fatty fish.

Fish's Nutrient Profile

Salmon, mackerel, and sardines are among the fatty fish that are rich in omega-3 fatty acids, which are good for the heart, the brain, and the control of inflammation.

Fish is a great source of high-quality protein and contains all the necessary amino acids.

Vitamins: Fish is a good source of vitamin D and some B vitamins, like B12.

Minerals: Iodine, which is necessary for thyroid function, and selenium are minerals found in fish.

Considerations

Variety: To ensure a balanced intake of nutrients, it's crucial to include a range of animal protein sources.

Lean vs. Fatty: Depending on your dietary preferences and goals, and taking into account your overall macronutrient balance, you can choose leaner cuts of meat or fattier cuts.

Sustainability: When deciding on sources of animal protein, take into account ethical issues like overfishing and animal farming practices.

A balanced diet should include a variety of foods to make sure you're getting all the vitamins, minerals, and nutrients your body needs for optimum health, even though animal protein sources are excellent sources of nutrients. You can make well-informed decisions by seeking the advice of a registered dietitian or healthcare professional based on your unique needs and goals.

Meat From Organs And Its Nutritional Value

The edible internal organs of animals are referred to as organ meats or offal. They have been valued for their rich nutrient content throughout history and have been consumed by many different cultures. They may not be as popular in modern diets, but because of their high nutrient density, they are a significant part of the Carnivore Diet and are regarded as nutritional powerhouses.

Organ meats come in a variety of forms, each with a distinctive nutrient profile. The liver, heart, kidneys, brain, tongue, and tripe (the lining of the stomach) are typical examples.

Organ meats are frequently more nutrient-dense than muscle meats in terms of nutritional value. They contain an abundance of vital vitamins, minerals, and other bioactive substances. Organ meats typically contain the following vitamins and minerals.

Vitamins: Organ meats are particularly high in vitamins, whereas muscle meats may be less vitamin-rich. For instance:

Vitamin A: The liver is a particularly excellent source of this vitamin, which is necessary for healthy skin, eyesight, and the immune system.

B vitamins: Different B vitamins, including B12, B6, riboflavin, and niacin, which are important for energy metabolism, the production of red blood cells, and the health of the nervous system, can be found in abundance in the liver, heart, and kidney.

Folate: Some organ meats, like the liver, contain a lot of folate, a necessary B vitamin crucial for DNA synthesis and cell division.

Minerals: Minerals like iron, zinc, selenium, and phosphorus are abundant in organ meats.

Heme iron, the kind of iron found in animal foods and essential for oxygen transport, is found in abundance in the liver, heart, and kidney. These organs are also good sources of heme iron.

Zinc: Organ meats are a good source of zinc, which helps with growth, wound healing, and immune function.

Selenium: Organ meats contain selenium, an antioxidant mineral.

Omega-3 fatty acids, which are present in brain tissue, are among the healthy fats found in some organ meats.

Benefits and Things to Think About

Satisfaction: The high nutrient content of organ meats can help people feel full longer and less frequently.

Cultural and ethical factors to consider Depending on the culture, eating organic meats can be a sustainable way to use more of the animal and minimize waste.

Organ meats are nutrient-rich, but it's still important to eat them in moderation and as part of a healthy diet. If consumed in large quantities, the high levels of some nutrients, such as vitamin A, copper, and iron, can cause an excessive intake. The acceptance of organ meats and their inclusion in the diet is also influenced by cultural and personal preferences.

Consult a registered dietitian or healthcare provider if you're interested in incorporating organ meats into your diet. They can assist you in figuring out the right serving sizes and making sure that your diet overall is balanced and meets your nutritional needs.

Dairy And Egg Products

Common animal-derived foods that offer a variety of nutrients and can be incorporated into the Carnivore Diet include dairy products and eggs. Although not technically "meat," these foods are still valuable sources of necessary nutrients and can add variety to a diet that primarily consists of animal products.

Products made from the milk of mammals like cows, goats, and sheep are known as dairy products. They span a variety of products like milk, cheese, yogurt, and butter.

Dairy products have a high nutritional value because they contain several important nutrients, including:

Calcium: Calcium, a mineral necessary for healthy bones,

muscles, and nerve transmission, is a well-known mineral found in dairy products.

Protein: Dairy products, particularly milk and cheese, offer a full source of protein that includes all necessary amino acids.

Vitamins: Riboflavin (B2), vitamin B12, and vitamin D are vitamins found in dairy products. Additionally, some products have extra vitamins added to them.

Fat: Different dairy products have different amounts of fat, including saturated fats in items like butter and full-fat dairy products.

Minerals: Dairy products provide phosphorus and magnesium, minerals that are crucial for bone health and several bodily processes.

Eggs: Eggs are a very nutrient-dense food that is also regarded as a complete protein source because they contain all nine essential amino acids. They are the reproductive organs that birds produce, with chicken eggs being the most widely consumed variety.

Eggs have a high nutritional value and offer a variety of necessary nutrients, including:

Protein: Eggs are a great option for people looking to meet their protein needs because they are a good source of high-quality protein.

Vitamins: Eggs are a good source of vitamins like riboflavin, vitamin D, and vitamin B12. They are also abundant in choline, which is crucial for the growth and health of the brain.

Healthy Fats: Eggs are a good source of omega-3 fatty acids and other healthy unsaturated fats, especially when they come from chickens raised on pasture.

Minerals: Minerals like phosphorus and selenium are present in eggs.

Considerations:

Lactose Intolerance/Dairy Allergies: These conditions can cause digestive discomfort in some people. Dairy products should either be avoided in such circumstances or consumed in a form that is better tolerated, such as lactose-free varieties.

Egg Allergies: Egg allergies are relatively common, and those who have them should stay away from eggs and foods that contain them.

Quality: Select high-quality sources when selecting dairy and egg products. Alternatives that are organic, pasture-raised, and free-range may have better nutrient profiles and be more environmentally sustainable.

Eggs and dairy products can be incorporated into a carnivore diet to increase dietary variety and provide additional nutrients. However, some people decide not to consume these foods because they come from plants (like eggs) or because they might contain allergens (like dairy).

As with any dietary decision, it's crucial to take into account your personal preferences, dietary requirements, and any existing medical conditions. A healthcare professional or registered dietitian can assist you in making knowledgeable choices about incorporating dairy products and eggs into your diet if you have specific dietary concerns or questions.

Chapter 4: Health Claims and Research

The Carnivore Diet and other low-carb, high-fat diets are frequently linked to outcomes like weight loss and changes in body composition. Here is a thorough explanation of how these changes take place, along with some things to think about:

1. **Loss of weight**

Through several mechanisms, the Carnivore Diet's emphasis on eating foods derived from animals while avoiding carbohydrates can promote weight loss:

Ketosis: The body enters a state of ketosis by significantly reducing the amount of carbohydrates it consumes. When in ketosis, the body primarily uses fat reserves as fuel rather than carbohydrates. Over time, this may cause a decrease in body fat.

Lower Calorie Intake: Many advocates of the Carnivore Diet claim to feel more satisfied and consume fewer calories. A calorie deficit, which is required for weight loss, can be produced as a result.

Control of Appetite: The high protein and fat content of the diet can aid in regulating appetite and lowering cravings, which can reduce instances of overeating.

2. Changes in Body Composition:
The ratio of lean body mass (muscle) to body fat can change as a result of the carnivore diet.

Lean Muscle Mass Preservation: Even during weight loss, the high protein content of the diet helps maintain lean muscle mass. To avoid muscle deterioration, it's critical to consume enough protein.

Fat Loss: The diet may cause weight loss by encouraging the use of fat for energy. Body fat percentage decreases as stored fat is broken down by the body.

Water weight: At first, individuals might lose weight quickly as a result of glycogen depletion. Restricting carbohydrates causes the body to release water that is stored with glycogen and decreases glycogen stores. This may result in a discernible loss of weight.

Factors to Bear in Mind

Individual Variability: Individual differences in weight loss and body composition can be attributed to a variety of factors, including genetics, metabolism, initial weight, and level of activity.

Effects in the Short vs. Long Term: As the body gets used to the low-carb diet, the initial rapid weight loss may slow down. It takes consistent dietary and lifestyle changes to manage weight over the long term.

Exercise and Muscle Mass: While a healthy diet may help people maintain their muscle mass, those who engage in resistance training or other high-intensity exercise may need to adjust their protein intake to promote muscle growth and recovery.

Nutrient Balance: While on the Carnivore Diet, it's essential to make sure you're still getting a variety of nutrients, vitamins, and minerals. Neglecting nutritional requirements in favor of weight loss can result in deficiencies.

Sustainability: The Carnivore Diet's long-term success depends on the individual's ability to maintain it. Extreme dietary restrictions can have an impact on adherence, mental health, and social interactions.

Monitoring and Consultation

It is advised to speak with a healthcare provider or registered dietitian before making any significant dietary changes to achieve weight loss or body composition goals. They can offer advice on how to maintain a balanced and sustainable approach to your dietary choices, help you set realistic goals, track your advancement, address potential nutrient deficiencies, and address these issues.

Regulation Of Blood Sugar And Insulin Sensitivity

In relation to the Carnivore Diet and other dietary philosophies, blood sugar control and insulin sensitivity are important aspects of metabolic health. Let's explore what they mean and how diet affects them:

Blood sugar control

The quantity of sugar (glucose) in the blood is referred to as blood sugar, also known as blood glucose. It serves as an essential source of fuel for the body's cells, especially the brain and muscles. However, general health must keep blood sugar levels stable.

The function of insulin

The pancreas secretes the hormone insulin, which is essential for controlling blood sugar levels. After consuming carbohydrates, the pancreas releases insulin into the bloodstream to lower blood sugar levels. Glucose absorption by cells is aided by insulin, which also lowers blood sugar levels.

Insensitivity to Insulin

The term "insulin sensitivity" describes how well cells react to insulin signals. Cells efficiently absorb glucose from the bloodstream in people with high insulin sensitivity, which contributes to stable blood sugar levels.

Carnivore diet and control of blood sugar:
The Carnivore Diet, which severely restricts carbohydrate consumption, can affect insulin sensitivity in a variety of ways.

Blood Sugar Levels Are Stable: Since the diet limits carbo-hydrates, blood sugar levels fluctuate less. Blood sugar stays largely constant without the peaks and valleys brought on by high-carb meals.

Less Need for Insulin: Since fewer carbohydrates are absorbed into the bloodstream, less insulin is required to help cells take up glucose. People who have type 2 diabetes or insulin resistance may benefit from this because it can reduce the amount of insulin secreted.

Weight loss and Insulin Sensitivity:
Reduced insulin resistance is frequently linked to weight loss. Insulin resistance and excess body weight are related, particularly to abdominal fat. Insulin sensitivity tends to increase with weight loss, making it simpler for cells to react to insulin signals.

Considerations:
While the Carnivore Diet may improve insulin sensitivity and blood sugar control, it's important to take other factors into account as well:

The balance of your nutrients should be maintained while keeping an eye out for any potential deficiency.

Different people react differently to dietary changes. The Carnivore Diet may help some people better regulate their blood sugar while having little to no effect on others.

Sustainability over the long term: The Carnivore Diet may be difficult to maintain over the long term, and it is still unknown how it may affect general health.

Monitoring and Consultation

Consult a healthcare provider if you are worried about how your blood sugar is regulated, your insulin sensitivity, or any other aspect of your metabolic health. You can manage your overall health by managing your blood sugar levels regularly and receiving advice from a registered dietitian or other healthcare professional.

Reduced inflammation

One of the potential advantages of the Carnivore Diet and other dietary regimens is that it may reduce inflammation, which is frequently mentioned. Understanding inflammation's potential effects on health—and how the diet might affect them—is essential.

Inflammation:

The immune system of the body naturally produces inflammation in response to injury, infection, or harmful stimuli. Immune cells are stimulated, specific molecules (like cytokines) are released, and blood flow to the affected area is increased. Acute inflammation aids in the body's healing process and is a temporary protective response. However, persistent inflammation known as chronic inflammation is linked to several health problems, including chronic diseases like diabetes, cardiovascular disease, and some autoimmune conditions.

Diet's Effect on Inflammation:
Inflammation is significantly influenced by diet. In the body, certain foods can either increase or decrease inflammation.

Dietary Carnivores and Inflammation
Inflammation may be decreased, according to proponents of the Carnivore Diet, by avoiding plant-based foods, especially those that contain substances that can elicit immune reactions. Here are some possible effects of inflammation on diet:

Avoiding anti-nutrients: Some plant substances, such as lectins and phytates found in grains and legumes, are regarded as anti-nutrients because they can obstruct the absorption of nutrients and may provoke immune reactions in susceptible people.

Potential for Gut Health: The Carnivore Diet's exclusion of plant fibers may be advantageous for people who struggle with specific digestive problems because fiber can occasionally aggravate the gut lining. Potentially, chronic inflammation could be decreased by improving the gut microbiome.

Considerations:
Although advocates of the Carnivore Diet assert that it lowers

inflammation, it's important to take the following things into account:

Nutrient Diversity: Cutting out plant foods may result in a lack of vitamins, minerals, and dietary fiber, all of which are crucial for maintaining overall health and controlling inflammation.

Balanced diet: Lifestyle, genetics, and environmental exposures are a few other factors besides diet that can affect inflammation. Usually, a balanced diet with a range of nutrient sources is advised.

Limited Research: The long-term effects of the Carnivore Diet and its influence on inflammation have received little attention from scientists. More thorough scientific research is required before making claims about reducing inflammation.

Monitoring and Consultation
   Consult a medical professional or registered dietitian before making any dietary changes to treat inflammation or other health issues. They can offer advice on managing inflammation through a balanced and evidence-based approach, assist you in making informed decisions, customize your diet to meet your unique needs, and more.

The Carnivore Diet and Autoimmune Conditions

Autoimmune disorders occur when the immune system, which is meant to defend the body against foreign invaders, inadvertently targets the body's healthy cells and tissues. Over 80 autoimmune diseases have been identified, including celiac disease, type 1 diabetes, lupus, multiple sclerosis, and rheumatoid arthritis. It's interesting to think about how the Carnivore Diet fits into the management of autoimmune disorders, but it's important to proceed carefully and take into account all the variables.

Chronic inflammation and autoimmune diseases:

Chronic inflammation is a defining characteristic of many autoimmune diseases. Inappropriate immune system attacks damage tissue and start inflammatory processes. Pain, exhaustion, and a decline in organ function are among the symptoms that these conditions frequently cause.

Dietary Carnivores and Autoimmune Diseases

Some people advocate the Carnivore Diet's exclusion of plant-based foods as a way to lessen autoimmune reaction triggers. Advocates claim that by avoiding plant substances like lectins, which may trigger immune reactions in sensitive people, the diet may help some people with autoimmune conditions.

Future Mechanisms

Elimination of Potential Triggers: Some plant substances, including lectins and particular grains, have been linked to the initiation or exacerbation of autoimmune reactions in vulnerable people. Limiting these substances in the diet might help to lessen inflammation.

Improved Gut Health: People with autoimmune conditions

that affect the gut may benefit from the diet's simplicity and lack of dietary fibers. Reduced inflammation may be a result of improved gut health.

Considerations:

Individual Variation: Autoimmune conditions are complicated, and the causes can differ greatly from person to person. One person's solution might not be suitable for another. It's important to listen to your body and seek medical advice.

Nutritional Balance: Although some people with autoimmune diseases may benefit from the Carnivore Diet, it also raises questions about nutrient deficiencies. To avoid nutrient imbalances, careful planning and potential supplementation are crucial.

Lack of Scientific Support: There is a dearth of studies examining the effects of the Carnivore Diet specifically for autoimmune disorders. Unknown are the diet's long-term effects, potential risks, and interactions with different autoimmune diseases.

Monitoring and Consultation

It's critical to follow a healthcare provider's advice when making dietary changes if you have an autoimmune condition. You can get advice from a registered dietitian or medical professional who can also make sure your nutritional needs are met and keep an eye on your health over time. It's important to prioritize a balanced approach to managing autoimmune conditions that takes into account medical advice, lifestyle factors, and general health even though some people may report improvements with the Carnivore Diet.

Considerations For Gut Microbiome And Digestive Health

The gut microbiome and digestive health are crucial for overall well being. It's interesting to learn how the Carnivore Diet affects gut health and the microbiome, but it's important to weigh the advantages and disadvantages of this diet.

Internal Health:
The term "digestive health" refers to the digestive system's proper operation, which includes breaking down food, absorbing nutrients, and getting rid of waste. The immune system, energy production, and nutrient absorption are all supported by a strong digestive system.

Stomach Microbiome

The diverse community of microorganisms that live in the digestive tract is referred to as the gut microbiome. These microbes—which include bacteria, viruses, fungi, and others—play an important part in metabolism, immune response, digestion, and even mental health.

Healthy Digestive System and Carnivore Diet:
The Carnivore Diet, which excludes plant-based foods, can affect digestive health in both favorable and unfavorable ways:
Positive Features
Potential for Symptom Relief: Some sufferers of gastroin-

testinal conditions like irritable bowel syndrome (IBS) or inflammatory bowel disease (IBD) claim that the Carnivore Diet has helped their symptoms. Some plant substances may cause gastrointestinal irritation, so their absence may lessen it.

Simpleness: For people with digestive sensitivities, the simplicity of the diet can make it simpler to identify trigger foods and manage symptoms.

Considerations:
   Fiber Absence: Dietary fiber, which is crucial for encouraging regular bowel movements, maintaining gut barrier function, and supporting the diversity of the gut microbiome, is not allowed on the Carnivore Diet.

Impact on the Microbiome: A lack of plant-based foods may result in a decreased intake of prebiotic fibers, which support good gut bacteria. The diversity and balance of the gut microbiome may be adversely impacted by this.

Considering Both Digestive Health and the Microbiome:

While the Carnivore Diet excludes plant-based foods, variety is important to ensure a range of nutrients and potential health benefits.

Supplements: Some people following the Carnivore Diet may need to think about taking supplements for specific nutrients and fiber replacements to support digestive health in the absence of plant foods.

Personalization: Digestive reactions vary greatly from person to person. Pay attention to your body's signals, and if you experience any digestive discomfort or worries, speak with a medical professional.

Chapter 5: Potential Risks and Controversies

Nutritional Deficiencies And Methods For Resolving Them

When your body doesn't get enough essential nutrients from your diet, nutrient deficiencies can happen, which can cause several health problems. Due to the Carnivore Diet's ban on plant-based foods, potential nutrient deficiencies are a concern. Following is a breakdown of typical nutrients that may be deficient in this diet and advice on how to address deficiencies:

1. **Vitamins**:

Vitamin C: Deficiency is a concern because the Carnivore Diet forbids the consumption of fruits and vegetables, which are the main sources of vitamin C. Immune system health, wound healing, and antioxidant defense all depend on vitamin C. Consider including small amounts of organ meats, which contain some vitamin C, such as liver or heart.

Without plant sources, vitamin A deficiency is possible, but animal-based foods, particularly liver, are high in preformed vitamin A (retinol), which is crucial for healthy vision, the immune system, and skin.

B vitamins: Animal foods are a great source of B vitamins like B12, riboflavin, and niacin. Good sources include organic meats, meat, and dairy goods. To ensure adequate intake, it's crucial to include a variety of these foods.

2. **Minerals**:
   Magnesium: Magnesium can be deficient in the Carnivore Diet and is present in many plant-based foods. Fish and shellfish are two examples of animal foods that are high in magnesium. You can also talk to a doctor about taking supplements.

Potassium: Plant foods are important sources of potassium, and the Carnivore Diet may cause a deficiency. Although some meat, seafood, and dairy products contain potassium, you may want to consider taking supplements or consulting a doctor.

3. **Fiber**:
   Dietary Fiber: Lack of plant fibers can affect gut health and bowel regularity. Traditional sources of fiber are not part of the Carnivore Diet, but some people take psyllium husk or other fiber supplements to keep their digestive systems in good shape.

4. Fatty Acids Omega-3

While fish is a good source of EPA and DHA, some people might not eat enough of it to meet their needs. To maintain heart and brain health, think about including fatty fish like salmon or taking fish oil supplements.

Nutrient Deficiencies Mitigation:

Diverse Animal Foods: Include a range of foods derived from animals, such as eggs, red meat, poultry, fish, and organ meats. This can guarantee a wider variety of nutrients.

Organ meats are particularly nutrient-dense and can fill in any vitamin and mineral deficiencies that may arise from consuming only muscle meats.

Supplementation: You may need to take supplements, depending on your dietary preferences and specific requirements. To choose the proper supplements and dosages, speak with a medical expert.

Monitoring regularly: Blood tests can help spot possible nutrient deficiencies. To determine your nutritional status and modify your diet or supplements as necessary, consult a healthcare professional.

Advising and Customization:

Consult a registered dietitian or other healthcare provider before starting any restrictive diet, including the Carnivore Diet. They can evaluate your specific nutritional requirements, assist you in addressing any deficiencies, and support you in making educated dietary decisions that will promote your overall health and well-being.

Impact On Cholesterol Levels And Heart Health

The effect of the Carnivore Diet on cholesterol levels and heart health is a hotly debated subject. Concerns about the diet's effects on cardiovascular health are raised by the emphasis it places on animal-based foods, especially those high in fat. An explanation of how the Carnivore Diet may affect cholesterol levels and heart health is provided below:

Heart health and the carnivore diet:

Potential Advantages

Weight Loss: The Carnivore Diet may improve heart health if it causes weight loss. A risk factor for cardiovascular disease is excess body weight.

Blood Sugar Regulation: People with type 2 diabetes or insulin resistance may benefit from the low-carbohydrate diet's ability to stabilize blood sugar levels.

Inflammation: Some supporters claim that eliminating plant-based compounds from the diet may help to reduce inflammation, which is a risk factor for cardiovascular disease.

Potential Disadvantages

Saturated Fats: The diet's emphasis on foods derived from

animals may lead to a high intake of saturated fats, which is linked to higher LDL cholesterol levels and a higher risk of heart disease.

Cholesterol Levels: Animal-based foods, especially fatty meat cuts, can increase LDL cholesterol levels, a cardiovascular disease risk factor.

Nutritional Balance: A lack of plant-based foods may result in deficiencies of nutrients that protect the heart, such as dietary fiber, antioxidants, and some vitamins.

Amounts of cholesterol

The Carnivore Diet's effect on cholesterol levels is one of the topics of the most heated debate:

LDL cholesterol is a component of total cholesterol, which some Carnivore Diet participants report having higher levels of.

HDL cholesterol is regarded as "good" cholesterol because it aids in removing extra cholesterol from the bloodstream. According to some studies, the diet may raise HDL cholesterol.

LDL Cholesterol: LDL cholesterol is referred to as "bad" cholesterol due to its association with a higher risk of heart disease. Saturated fat consumption from the diet may cause some people to have higher LDL cholesterol levels.

Various Reactions:

The way each person reacts to dietary changes varies greatly. The Carnivore Diet may have positive effects for some people while having negative effects for others.

Monitoring and Consultation

Consult a medical professional before beginning the Carnivore Diet or making any dietary changes, especially if you want to improve your heart health. It's crucial to routinely monitor blood pressure, cholesterol levels, and other heart health indicators. A registered dietitian can assist you in navigating the diet's potential advantages and disadvantages and can collaborate with you to create a balanced strategy that supports your objectives for heart health. Prioritizing an individualized strategy that takes into account all cardiovascular risk factors as well as medical advice is crucial.

Sustainability And Viability Over The Long Term

When assessing the potential of the Carnivore Diet as a dietary approach, it is crucial to take its long-term viability and feasibility into account. Long-term diet adoption necessitates careful consideration of feasibility, nutritional balance, and general well-being.

1. Nutritional Suitability:

Making sure a diet contains all the essential nutrients required for good health is part of sustainability. Due to the exclusion of plant-based foods, the Carnivore Diet's restrictive nature raises questions about possible nutrient deficiencies. Following a diet that consistently lacks essential vitamins, minerals, fiber, and antioxidants can eventually result in health problems.

2. Diverse Nutrients:

To ensure a wide variety of nutrients, a sustainable diet needs to include a variety of foods. Due to its heavy reliance on animal products, the Carnivore Diet may have a limited range of nutrients, which could result in a lack of certain vitamins, minerals, and other beneficial compounds found in plant foods.

3. Bowel Health:

By reducing the variety of helpful gut bacteria, a diet low in dietary fiber and prebiotics from plant foods can hurt gut health. Better overall health is linked to a gut microbiome with a variety of bacteria.

4. Psychological and social influences:

Sustainability also involves taking into account a diet's social and psychological components. The Carnivore Diet's stringent restrictions may have an impact on how people interact with one another, observe cultural customs, and enjoy their food. It's important to remember that eating has both mental and emotional components.

5. Practicality:

A sustainable diet should be feasible to maintain while traveling, eating out, and participating in social activities. It may be difficult to navigate these situations without problems due to the Carnivore Diet's strict restrictions.

6. Long-Term Health Consequences:

The long-term health effects of the Carnivore Diet are not well understood, even though short-term studies and anecdotes suggest potential benefits. Over a long period, the absence of plant-based foods may have unanticipated effects on health outcomes.

7. Personalization:

Genetics, metabolism, medical conditions, and other factors, among others, can greatly affect how each person reacts to diets. Personalization is crucial for long-term success because what works for one person may not work for another.

8. professional direction

Consult a registered dietitian or other healthcare professional before beginning the Carnivore Diet or any other restrictive diet for a prolonged period. They can support you in overcoming obstacles, advise on nutrient intake, keep an eye on your health, and make sure that your dietary decisions are in line with your long-term health objectives.

The Carnivore Diet may, in the short term, benefit some people, but its sustainability and viability over the long term raise serious questions. To promote general health and well-being, a well-rounded, balanced diet that contains a variety of nutrient sources, including plant foods, is typically advised. Prioritize a diet that you can stick to comfortably over the long term, one that satisfies your nutritional requirements and fosters a positive relationship with food.

Environmental And Ethical Issues

Any diet, including the Carnivore Diet, should be evaluated in light of ethical and environmental issues. These factors include how dietary decisions affect ecosystems, animals, and sustainability.

Ethical Issues

Animal Welfare: Concerns about the moral treatment of animals in agriculture are raised by the Carnivore Diet's emphasis on animal products. Some people view industrial farming methods, which can include confinement and the use of antibiotics, as unethical.

Use of Animal Products: Because so many foods in the diet come from animals, there may be a rise in the demand for animal farming. Large-scale animal agriculture has ethical and environmental repercussions, which raise ethical questions.

Plant-based Ethical Views: For people who place a high priority on moral issues when making food decisions, the diet's exclusion of plant-based foods may run counter to their moral principles. For the sake of sustainability and lessening the harm done to animals, many people choose plant-based diets.

Environmental Issues

Carbon Footprint: Meat production on a large scale and animal agriculture in general both contribute to greenhouse gas emissions. Compared to diets based primarily on plants, an animal-product-focused diet may have a larger carbon footprint.

Land Use and Deforestation: Growing livestock requires a sizable amount of both land and water. Deforestation can take place to make grazing land or grow crops for animal feed, which results in habitat loss and a decline in biodiversity.

Water Use: Meat production uses significantly more water than plant-based food production, making animal agriculture a water-intensive industry.

Biodiversity: Animal agriculture's effects on ecosystems may result in a loss of biodiversity and the disruption of natural habitats.

Ethical and Sustainable Decisions:

Reduced Meat Consumption: For those worried about the moral and environmental consequences, cutting back on meat consumption and opting for animal products from sustainably sourced sources can be a compromise.

Plant-based substitutes: Including more plant-based foods in your diet can help you live more ethically and leave a smaller environmental footprint.

Local and organic: When possible, choose locally sourced and organic animal products to support farming methods that emphasize animal welfare and sustainability.

Learn about farming practices, sourcing strategies, and food labels to empower yourself to make decisions that are in line with your values.

Make wise decisions:

The ethical and environmental ramifications of any diet, including the Carnivore Diet, should be taken into account in addition to health considerations. Making dietary decisions that are consistent with your values and that advance your general well-being can be aided by balancing personal preferences, health objectives, ethical considerations, and environmental impact. Making informed decisions can be facilitated by consulting with experts, such as registered dietitians and environmental organizations.

social and psychological aspects

When assessing the Carnivore Diet's potential effects on general well-being, it is crucial to take its psychological and social components into account. These factors include social interactions, the connection between food and mental health, and the possible negative effects of dietary restrictions on emotional and mental states.

Psychiatric considerations

Food and Mood: What we eat can affect our mental and emotional well-being. Serotonin levels may be impacted by restrictive diets like the Carnivore Diet, which could affect mood regulation.

Food enjoyment: Pleasure and cultural experiences are frequently connected to food. The variety and enjoyment of meals may be restricted by a restrictive diet, potentially affecting overall satisfaction.

Orthorexia: The Carnivore Diet's stringent dietary guidelines may be a contributing factor in orthorexic tendencies, a fixation on "clean" eating that can result in obsession and anxiety.

Social Factors

Sharing meals with others is a social activity. A restrictive diet may make it difficult to interact with others, attend events, or eat out.

Cultural and religious considerations: Cultural and religious beliefs can have an impact on dietary decisions. These values might be at odds with a diet that eliminates particular foods.

Family dynamics may be impacted by a restrictive diet, particularly if other family members have different dietary preferences.

Health and well-being must be balanced.

Personal Values: Take into account how your dietary preferences fit with your values and level of wellness. Give both mental and physical health a top priority.

Moderation: Dieting to extremes can have an impact on mental health. To promote balance and overall enjoyment, moderation, and variety in food choices are beneficial.

Flexibility: Maintain a balance between your dietary objectives and your ability to adapt to social situations and cultural customs. A wider variety of foods can occasionally be incorporated to aid in navigating social situations.

Support from professionals: If you're having trouble with the psychological aspects of food and diet, you might want to talk to a mental health professional or a registered dietitian who focuses on disordered eating.

Mindful Eating:

Developing mindful eating habits can assist with navigating psychological and social issues:

Pay attention to your body's signals of hunger and fullness. Instead of focusing on outside rules, consider internal signals.

Enjoyment: Cherish the flavors of your meals and value the dining experience.

Emotional Awareness: Be aware of the emotions that cause changes in your eating habits and look into healthier coping mechanisms.

Self-compassion: Be compassionate with your dietary decisions. Avoid negative self-talk and self-criticism.

In conclusion, it is crucial to take into account the psychological and social effects of the Carnivore Diet when assessing its potential effects. Making dietary decisions that support holistic wellness requires striking a balance between physical and mental health, taking pleasure in social interactions, and upholding a healthy relationship with food.

Chapter 6: Getting Started on the Carnivore Diet

Mentally Preparing And Establishing Reasonable Expectations

When considering any dietary change, including the Carnivore Diet, mental preparation and the setting of reasonable expectations are essential steps. By taking these actions, you can make sure that your mind is set up for any challenges and adjustments that may come up during the transition and afterward.

1. **Become Informed**

Do your homework and learn everything you can about the Carnivore Diet's guiding principles, potential advantages, and drawbacks. Recognize the scientific basis for various dietary stances.

2. **Set Specific Goals**

Determine your specific health objectives before considering a carnivore diet. Having clear intentions can help direct your journey, whether it involves losing weight, managing a health condition, or achieving other goals.

3. **Setting realistic goals**

Recognize that results in the short term may not be the same as those in the long term. Initial weight loss or other changes might not be long-term sustainable.

Recognize that progress isn't necessarily linear and that it could be uneven. Although plateaus and setbacks can occur, persistence and patience are essential.

4. **Mental Readiness:**

Develop an optimistic and receptive mindset. Accept the diet as an experiment and be prepared to change it as your body changes.

Addressing Obstacles: Be aware of potential obstacles like social situations, cravings, and emotional setbacks. Create a plan of action to overcome these obstacles without getting too overwhelmed.

Flexibility: Be ready to change your strategy in response to your body's signals and how you are feeling. With flexibility, you can modify the diet to suit your needs.

5. **Balanced Methodology:**

Strive for variety within the parameters of the Carnivore Diet if you decide to follow it. Include various animal products and experiment with various cooking techniques.

Intake of Nutrients: Emphasize consuming a variety of nutrients. To address any potential deficiencies, take into account supplementation.

6. **Advice from Professionals**:

Consult experts: Before beginning any diet, speak with registered dietitians and members of the medical community. They can address your concerns, offer specialized advice, and assist you in making well-informed decisions.

7. **Watch and Think:**

Self-Reflection: Consider how your health, energy, mood, and general well-being are being affected by your diet regularly. Be willing to modify your plans in light of your experiences.

Pay Attention to Your Body:

Body Signals: Be aware of your energy levels, hunger cues, and body signals. Trust the advice from your body.

9. **Mental Well-Being:**

Emotional Well-Being: Take into account how the diet will affect your emotional state. Reevaluate the diet's suitability for your mental health if you discover that it is causing you distress or unpleasant feelings.

In conclusion, when considering the Carnivore Diet or any dietary change, mental preparation and realistic expectations are crucial. You can navigate the difficulties and ambiguities that may surface during your dietary journey by taking a balanced and knowledgeable approach, as well as having self-awareness and adaptability. Always put your overall health, including your physical and mental well-being, first.

Starting The Diet In Transition

To help your body adjust to the new way of eating, transitioning to the Carnivore Diet necessitates careful planning, preparation, and a gradual approach. Here is a step-by-step tutorial for starting the diet:

1. **Education and research**
   Learn about the Carnivore Diet's guiding principles, permitted foods, potential advantages, and potential drawbacks.

2. **Professional consultation**:
   Medical Advice: Speak with a doctor before making any major dietary changes, especially if you have any pre-existing conditions.

Consider working with a registered dietitian who can offer individualized advice and assist you in organizing a balanced transition.

3. **Setting up:**
   Stock up on a variety of animal-based foods like beef, poultry, fish, eggs, and organ meats as well as other kitchen necessities.

Supplements: Talk to a medical expert about whether you need to take any supplements to make up for any potential nutrient deficiencies.

4. Gradual Change:

Reduce Carbohydrates: Gradually cut back on the amount of grains, fruits, and starchy vegetables that are high in carbohydrates.

Transition to Animal Foods: Begin consuming more animal products while progressively reducing your intake of plant foods. Introduce fattier cuts gradually after starting with leaner meats.

Water and other non-caloric beverages can help you stay hydrated.

5. Pay attention to your body's signals:

Physical signals: Be aware of how your body reacts to the adjustments. Be aware of adjustments to your energy levels, digestion, and general well-being.

6. Modification and adaptation:

Digestive Adaptation: During the transition, some people go through digestive changes. Consider including foods that are easier on your stomach and give your body time to adjust.

7. Variety in Food:

Investigate Various Animal Foods: To ensure a wider range of nutrients, gradually introduce a variety of animal-based foods.

8. Tracking Nutritional Intake:

Obtain a variety of nutrients, such as vitamins, minerals, and essential fatty acids, to ensure that your diet is balanced. To create a balanced meal plan, consult a registered dietitian if necessary.

9. **Electrolytes and Hydration:**

Sodium and electrolytes: Your body's electrolyte balance may change as you transition. Consuming enough sodium can help stop electrolyte imbalances.

Support for Social and Emotional Needs:

10. **Social Situations**: Discuss your dietary changes and any potential difficulties with friends and family members when you are out and about.

Your emotional health is important. Be mindful of it. If the diet makes you feel bad or upset, think about changing your strategy.

11. **Gradual Modification**:

Patience: Give your body enough time to get used to the new eating habits. Sometimes progress isn't quick or straightforward.

12. **Consistent Monitoring**:

Examine your health, your level of energy, and any changes in how you feel regularly. If you have any worries, speak with a medical expert.

13. **Seek Advice from a Professional:**

Registered Dietitian: To make sure your nutritional needs are met and your health goals are supported, think about obtaining ongoing advice from a registered dietitian.

The Carnivore Diet must be adopted gradually, taking into account your unique needs and current state of health. Making small, gradual changes while paying attention to your body and, as necessary, consulting a professional are the keys. Keep in mind that the transition is a process, and throughout the journey, you should put your general well-being first.

Preparing Meals And Recipes

For the Carnivore Diet to be successful, meal planning and recipes are crucial. You can ensure that you're getting the nutrition you need while still enjoying your food by planning balanced and varied meals. To plan meals and find recipes that are appropriate for the carnivore diet, follow these steps:

Meal preparation:

Prioritize Variety in Nutrients

To make sure you're getting a variety of nutrients, try to include a variety of animal-based foods.

Include a variety of animal foods

To diversify your nutrient intake, include red meat (beef, lamb), poultry (chicken, turkey), fish, organ meats, and eggs.

Think about Nutrient Density

Choose foods that are high in nutrients, such as organ meats, which are loaded with vitamins and minerals.

Scheduled Portion:

To satisfy both your nutritional and energy needs, balance your portion sizes.

Hydration:

Water and other calorie-free beverages can help you stay hydrated.

Observe the electrolytes:

To keep a healthy balance, watch your sodium and other electrolyte intake.

Supplements:

To ascertain whether you require any supplements to make up for potential deficiencies, speak with a healthcare professional.

Recipe Concepts:

Beef or Steak Patties
Season steak or ground beef patties with salt and pepper before cooking.
Grilled turkey or chicken

You can season chicken breasts or turkey cutlets on the grill to your liking.
Sloppy Fish.

For omega-3 fatty acids, eat fatty fish like salmon, mackerel, or sardines.
  Eggs.

Cook eggs in a variety of ways, including fried, scrambled, boiled, or poached.
  Animal Organs.

Try liver, heart, and kidney meats, which are rich in nutrients.
  Bone broths and broths.

Utilize connective tissues and bones to create nutrient-rich broths.
  Vegetarian Stews.

Use bone broth and meat to make stews, and for flavor, add herbs and spices.
  Burgers for carnivores.

From ground beef, form patties and season to taste.
  Delights wrapped in bacon.

To add flavor, wrap meat or organ meats in bacon.
  grilled seafood

In a skillet, sear shrimp, scallops, or other seafood.

Resources for Recipes

The Carnivore Diet is promoted on websites and blogs that

provide a variety of recipes and meal suggestions.

Recipe ideas could come from books and cookbooks that are devoted to carnivore or ketogenic diets.

Personalization:

Recipes should be modified to fit your culinary preferences, dietary restrictions, and cultural requirements. To keep your meals interesting and satisfying, experiment with different meat cuts, cooking techniques, and seasonings.

Planning and Consultations:

Consider working with a registered dietitian if you're new to the Carnivore Diet or if you need assistance with meal planning. They can offer guidance, address nutritional concerns, and assist you in planning well-balanced meals to make sure your diet supports your health objectives while satisfying your nutrient requirements.

Potential Problems And Strategies For Solving Them

Like any dietary strategy, the Carnivore Diet has potential drawbacks of its own. For the diet to be successful, it is essential to be aware of these difficulties and have solutions ready. The following are some typical problems with the carnivore diet and solutions for them:

1. Lack of certain nutrients

Problem: Avoiding plant-based foods may result in vitamin, mineral, and fiber deficiencies.

Include nutrient-dense animal foods like organ meats and fatty cuts as a solution. If recommended by a medical professional, think about taking supplements.

2. Social Context:

Challenge: Eating out and attending social events can be difficult when you follow a strict diet.

Solution: Let your loved ones know about your dietary preferences. Whenever you go out to eat, order meat-based dishes or bring your food.

3. Digestive Modifications

Problem: Making the switch to a high-meat diet can result in digestive changes like constipation or alterations in bowel habits.

Solution: Introduce new foods gradually and track your body's reactions. Increase your water intake and think about adding bone broth or other gastrointestinal-friendly foods.

4. Cravings and Mental Health Issues:

Problem: Dietary restrictions may cause psychological problems such as food cravings for familiar foods.

Solution: Eat mindfully and satisfy cravings by deciding on nutrient-dense animal foods. Keep your attention on the potential advantages that inspired you to try the diet.

5. **Cooking Exhaustion:**

Problem: Relying too heavily on animal products may cause you to get bored or tired of cooking.

Solution: To keep your meals interesting and tasty, experiment with various meat cuts, cooking techniques, and seasonings.

6. **Sustainability over time:**

Long-term adherence to a strict diet can be difficult due to its lack of variety.

Solution: To avoid nutrient deficiencies, think about reintroducing a wider variety of foods. Adopt a more accommodating diet that permits occasional consumption of plant-based foods.

7. **Social Exclusion:**

Having trouble attending social events because of dietary restrictions.

Solution: Inform your loved ones about your dietary preferences. Look for encouraging online groups where you can meet people who have similar diets.

8. **Travel Navigation:**

Maintaining a healthy diet while traveling can be challenging, especially in locations with few food options.

Plan and bring transportable, shelf-stable foods made of animal products. Look into nearby restaurants and options that provide suitable options.

9. **Environmental and sustainability issues:**
   Problem: A diet that prioritizes animal products may conflict with ethical and environmental concerns.

Solution: Make educated decisions by choosing sustainably sourced animal products and, when practical, incorporating plant-based alternatives.

10. **Managing Intake of Nutrients:**

Challenge: Without careful planning, obtaining a balanced nutrient intake can be difficult.

Solution: To make sure you're meeting your nutritional needs, speak with a registered dietitian. Create menus with a range of animal foods.

Keep in mind that every person's experiences are unique, so what works for one person may not work for another. Prioritize your health and well-being, and change your diet as necessary to fit your preferences and goals. A registered dietitian or healthcare professional can offer personalized advice to address potential challenges and ensure a safe and balanced approach if you're thinking about trying the carnivore diet.

Chapter 7: Personalizing The Carnivore Diet

Variations Within The Strict Versus Modified Carnivore Diet

There are various variations of the Carnivore Diet that people may adopt depending on their preferences, health objectives, and beliefs. The strict carnivore diet and the modified or flexible carnivore diet are the two main variations. An explanation of each follows:

1. A strictly carnivorous diet

The strict carnivore diet, also known as the "zero-carb" or "all-meat" diet, calls for the exclusion of all plant-based foods, such as grains, legumes, fruits, and vegetables in favor of the consumption of only animal-based foods. The primary emphasis is on nutrient sources derived from animals, such as:

Red meat, poultry, and seafood are all types of meat.

Organ Meats: Organ meats that are high in nutrients, such as liver, heart, and kidney.

Eggs: Both egg yolks and whites are acceptable.

Dairy: Due to their lactose content, some strict carnivores may consume dairy products like butter and cheese.

2. A flexible or modified carnivore diet

By including some plant-based foods or allowing for different food options, the modified or flexible carnivore diet allows for some degree of flexibility. People who want to reap the benefits of the diet while addressing potential nutrient deficiencies or moral concerns may prefer this version. The altered carnivore diet may consist of:

Low-carb vegetables like spinach or avocado are examples of limited plant foods. Other people include small amounts of other plant foods, such as those high in antinutrients and carbohydrates.

The cyclic approach alternates between strict carnivore eating and reintroducing small amounts of plant foods.

Considerations:

Personalization: Individual preferences, health objectives, and food tolerance can all be taken into account when creating either variation.

Nutrient Diversity: While a strict carnivore diet may eventually result in nutrient deficiencies, a modified version that includes some plant foods may offer a more balanced nutrient intake.

A strict animal-based diet raises concerns about ethics and the environment, which the modified version can help to address.

Trial and Error: To find the Carnivore Diet balance and variation that is best for your body and goals, you may have to experiment a little.

Professional Advice: It is advised to speak with a registered dietitian or other healthcare provider if you are thinking about implementing any variation of the carnivore diet. They can offer you individualized advice and make sure that your dietary decisions support your health requirements and objectives.

In conclusion, the Carnivore Diet offers a variety of adaptations to suit different preferences and objectives. No matter if you adopt a strict carnivore diet or a modified one, it's crucial to emphasize eating a healthy, balanced diet that meets your nutritional needs and promotes your overall well being.

Timing Of Meals And Intermittent Fasting

Some people use the Carnivore Diet in conjunction with strategies like meal planning and intermittent fasting (IF) to maximize its potential health benefits. Cycles of eating and fasting occur during intermittent fasting. The specific times of day that you eat your meals are referred to as meal timing. Here is a description of both ideas and how the Carnivore Diet relates to them.

IF: Intermittent Fasting

Instead of being a particular diet, intermittent fasting is an eating pattern. There are several well-liked IF techniques:

The 16/8 Method entails 16 hours of fasting and an 8-hour window for eating. You might, for instance, eat between 12:00 and 8:00 p.m. and observe a fast from 8:00 to 12:00 p.m. the following day.

The 5:2 Method entails eating normally five days a week while significantly reducing calorie intake (typically between 500 and 600 calories) on the other two days that are not consecutive.

Alternate-Day Fasting: This strategy alternates between eating days and fasting days (either complete fasting or very low-calorie intake).

Eat-Stop-Eat: This involves going without food for one or two days a week.

Warrior Diet: This entails eating a single large meal at night and small amounts of raw fruits and vegetables during the day.

Eating Period:

The distribution of meals throughout the day is referred to as meal timing. To maximize their results while following the Carnivore Diet, some people select particular meal timing techniques:

One or Two Meals: Some people find it more satisfying to eat one or two larger meals throughout their eating window.

The timing of meals and nutrient intake can support muscle growth and recovery if protein intake is timed to coincide with workouts.

Combining the Carnivore Diet and Intermittent Fasting:

Controlling one's appetite is a benefit of intermittent fasting, which may be helpful when consuming the filling meals recommended by the Carnivore Diet.

Fasting can increase metabolic flexibility, making it easier for the body to switch between using glucose and fats for energy.

Improved insulin sensitivity brought on by IF may aid in controlling blood sugar levels.

Longer fasting intervals can trigger autophagy, a cellular process that eliminates damaged cells and promotes general health.

Considerations:

Personalization: Depending on a person's preferences and reactions, intermittent fasting and meal timing may or may not be effective.

Gradual Adaptation: Start IF or meal timing gradually if you're a beginner to give your body time to adjust.

Professional Advice: Before attempting intermittent fasting, especially in conjunction with a specialized diet like the Carnivore Diet, consult a healthcare professional if you have underlying health conditions.

Individual responses may differ, but incorporating intermittent fasting and optimizing meal timing can be useful strategies to support the Carnivore Diet. For general success, paying attention to your body, staying hydrated, and getting a balanced diet are still crucial.

Adjusting The Diet For Particular Health Conditions And Goals

The Carnivore Diet can be customized to address unique needs, preferences, and medical considerations to meet specific health goals and conditions. Here are some ways to modify the Carnivore Diet for various health conditions and goals:

1. Loss of Weight:
   Focus on Protein: Give protein-rich foods top priority to support satiety and muscle maintenance.
   Keep an eye on Portion Sizes: To lose weight, keep an eye on your calorie intake.
   Hydration: Drink plenty of water to promote satiety and metabolism.
   Limit dairy and fat intake if you're trying to lose weight. Also, cut back on high-fat meat cuts.

2. Gaining muscle:

Increased Protein Intake: Eat enough protein to support the synthesis of muscle protein.

Diverse Protein Sources: To provide a range of amino acids, use a variety of animal protein sources.

Post-Workout Nutrition: To speed up recovery, eat a protein-rich meal after working out.

3: Blood sugar control:

Protein should be prioritized to reduce blood sugar spikes.

Watch Your Fat Intake: Keep an eye on your fat intake because too much of it can affect your insulin sensitivity.

Avoid Sugars: Sugars are naturally avoided because the diet doesn't include any carbohydrates.

4. Autoimmune Disorders:

Elimination Diet;To find potential trigger foods, think of the Carnivore Diet as an elimination diet.

Work with a healthcare professional to identify specific trigger foods if necessary. Food Sensitivity Testing.

Concentrate on Nutrient Density: For nutrient support, include organ meats and fatty fish.

5: Intestinal Health:

Introduce new foods gradually to prevent digestive discomfort during the transition.

Stay hydrated and keep your electrolyte levels balanced for good digestive health.

Include Bone Broth: Bone broth can aid in digestive health and gut healing.

6. Mood and Hormones:
Balanced nutrient intake: Make sure you're getting enough nutrients, such as micronutrients and essential fats.
Avoid Too Much Fat: Avoid consuming cuts of meat with a lot of fat because they might mess with your hormone balance.

8. Mental Well-Being:
Include fatty fish to get your omega-3s, which may help with brain health.
Balanced Nutrient Intake: To support mental health, make sure that your overall nutrient intake is balanced.
Consult Experts: If diet has an impact on your mood or general well-being, seek advice from mental health professionals.

9. Particular Health Conditions:
Consultation: To tailor the diet to particular medical conditions, collaborate with healthcare professionals, including registered dietitians.
Consider taking the recommended supplements to make up for any potential nutrient deficiencies.

10. Environmental and ethical issues:

Flexibility: Within the Carnivore Diet, choose ethically sourced animal products and investigate plant-based alternatives.
Choose animal products that are locally and sustainably produced.

11. Sustainability Over Time:
Moderation and Variety: To ensure long-term nutrient diversity, gradually reintroduce plant-based foods.

Flexible Approach: To accommodate long-term sustainability, take into account a modified or cyclical approach.

To tailor the Carnivore Diet to particular health goals and conditions, keep in mind that individual responses vary and that consulting with healthcare professionals is essential. The objective is to develop a personalized, well-balanced approach that promotes general health and well-being.

Chapter 8: Monitoring and Optimizing Health

Importance Of Regular Checkups And Medical Supervision

When considering any specialized diet, including the Carnivore Diet, medical supervision and routine checkups are essential. Here's why they're crucial:

1. Personalized Advice

Health Assessment: A medical expert can evaluate your current health, medical history, and any underlying conditions that might make it risky for you to follow the Carnivore Diet.

Personalization: A healthcare professional can adjust dietary advice to fit your unique health requirements, objectives, and potential restrictions.

2. **Nutrient equilibrium**

A healthcare professional can assist you in preventing any nutrient deficiencies that could result from cutting out particular food groups.

Supplements: If necessary, a healthcare professional can suggest the right supplements to fill in any nutrient gaps.

3. **Health Observation:**

Regular Check-Ups: Routine medical examinations can help you keep track of changes in your health and identify any potential problems before they become serious.

Blood tests: Blood tests can reveal information about your blood sugar, cholesterol, and other health markers, as well as your nutrient and nutrient levels. These tests can aid in locating any risks or imbalances.

4. **Taking Care of Medical Conditions**

A healthcare professional can advise you on how the diet might impact your condition and help you modify your approach if you have a chronic health condition (such as diabetes, heart disease, or autoimmune disorders).

Management of Medication: Some medical conditions call for the use of medication, and dietary changes may have an impact on how well a medication is metabolized. Safe management is ensured by medical supervision.

5. **Progress Monitoring:**

Weight and Body Composition: To make sure that your weight and body composition changes are in line with your goals and health, a healthcare professional can assist you in keeping track of these changes.

Physical and Mental Well-Being: You can talk about any physical or mental changes you've had since beginning the diet at regular check-ins.

6. **Resolving Issues**

A healthcare professional can assist you in understanding and managing any side effects that may develop as you switch to the diet.

If you experience changes or discomfort in your digestion, they can offer advice.

7. **Avoiding Harm**

Avoiding Extreme Measures: Medical supervision helps prevent extreme measures, such as excessive restriction or nutrient imbalances, that could be harmful to your health.

Risk Mitigation: A medical professional can advise you on how to adhere to the diet safely and reduce potential risks.

Long-Term Wellness:

Sustainability: A healthcare professional can assist you in determining whether the diet is sustainable and beneficial to your long-term health objectives.

9. **Monitoring Environmental and Ethical Issues:**

Balanced Approach: If ethical and environmental issues are significant to you, a healthcare professional can assist you in balancing these issues with your medical requirements.

In conclusion, when considering the Carnivore Diet or any specialized dietary approach, medical supervision and regular checkups are imperative. They make sure you're safe, address any health risks, give you individualized advice, and support you in making choices that are in line with your general well-being. Before making significant dietary changes, it is strongly advised to consult with medical professionals such as doctors and registered dietitians.

Tracking Important Health Indicators (blood tests, physical measurements)

When adhering to the Carnivore Diet or any dietary plan, it is crucial to keep track of important health indicators like blood work and body measurements. Monitoring these markers offers useful information about your health, development, and any potential problem areas. Here's how to monitor these important health indicators effectively:

1. Blood Tests

Blood tests can help you spot any changes or imbalances by giving you information about how your body is internally operating. Among the significant milestones to monitor are:

Levels of cholesterol can offer information about cardiovascular health, including total cholesterol, HDL (high-density lipoprotein), LDL (low-density lipoprotein), and triglycerides.

Blood Sugar Levels: Blood sugar control indicators include fasting blood glucose and HbA1c.

Track the levels of vitamins (such as B12 and D), minerals (such as iron), and other vital nutrients to look for deficiencies.

C-reactive protein (CRP) and ESR (erythrocyte sedimentation rate) are examples of inflammation markers.

Liver and Kidney Function: Tests like creatinine and liver enzymes can be used to determine how well these organs are functioning.

2. Body Dimensions:

Monitoring changes in body composition and general health can be done tangibly by tracking body measurements:

Weight: To keep track of changes in body weight, weigh yourself frequently.

Body Composition: To keep track of changes in muscle and fat mass, think about using instruments like skinfold calipers, DEXA scans, or scales that measure body fat percentage.

Measure your waist circumference to keep tabs on changes in abdominal fat.

3. How to Follow:

Before making dietary changes, start by getting baseline blood-work and body measurements. This offers a foundation for contrast.

Schedule routine check-ups with medical professionals to keep track of how your health indicators change over time.

Your doctor may advise how frequently to perform blood tests and measure body metrics, depending on your health objectives and any existing conditions.

Consistency: To ensure accurate tracking, use the same techniques and settings each time you take a measurement, such as using the same scale and similar lighting conditions to determine body weight.

4. Interpreting the Findings

Work with medical professionals, such as registered dietitians and doctors, to interpret measurements and blood work in the context of your overall health.

Trends Over Time: Instead of concentrating solely on individual values, look for trends in your health markers. Over time, consistent changes are more instructive.

5. Making Modifications:

Changes in Health Markers: If you notice any significant changes in your health markers, talk to your doctor to see if your diet needs to be changed.

Addressing Concerns: If you find areas that need attention, work with a healthcare expert to find dietary adjustments, lifestyle adjustments, or medical interventions to address them.

6. Holistic Strategy:

Keep in mind that health has many facets, and while blood tests and measurements are crucial, they should also be taken into account along with other aspects of well-being like energy levels, mood, digestion, and general well-being.

In conclusion, keeping track of important health indicators like blood work and body measurements gives you a complete picture of your health and how the Carnivore Diet is working for you. It's important to regularly monitor your health and consult with medical experts to make sure you're making decisions that will support your general well-being.

Modifying The Diet Based On Each Person's Response

The Carnivore Diet must be modified based on individual responses to maximize your experience and results. People's bodies can react to dietary changes in various ways, so it's important to pay attention to your own body's signals and make the necessary adjustments. Following are some effective diet modifications based on personal responses:

1: Pay Attention to Your Body:
  Physical signs: Keep track of how your body changes in response to the diet. Take note of any changes in your mood, digestion, energy level, and general well-being.

2. Gradual Alterations:
  Transition Period: Recognize that it might take some time for your body to adjust to the new eating habits. Introduce new foods gradually while keeping an eye on your feelings.

3. Recognize Positive and Negative Shifts:
  Positive Reactions: Pay attention to any improvements, like increased vigor, mental clarity, better digestion, or weight loss.

Negative Reactions: Pay attention to any unfavorable alterations, such as gastrointestinal discomfort, energy slumps, or adjustments in sleeping habits.

4. Overcoming Obstacles:
  Digestive Distress: If you have digestive distress, you might

want to change the kinds of animal foods you're eating or the way they're prepared.

Energy Levels: If you experience changes in your energy levels, consider your meal frequency and variety.

5. Potential Modifications:
   To ensure a wider range of nutrients, increase the variety of animal foods.

Meal Timing: Try eating at various times of the day to see if it affects your digestion or energy levels.

Change the proportions of proteins, fats, and carbohydrates to see how they affect your health.

Include Plant Foods: If you're using a flexible carnivore approach and find that consuming small amounts of low-carb plant foods improves your health, you might want to do so.

6. Consult with experts:
   Healthcare Providers: Consult with medical professionals like doctors or registered dietitians if you're going through a lot of negative changes or are worried about how the diet is affecting your health.

7. Maintain Records
   Keep a thorough record of your meals, how you feel after eating, and any obvious changes in your body in your food diary.

8. Flexibility is Important:
   Trial and Error: It may take some trial and error to find the ideal balance. Be willing to try out various strategies.

9. Keep an eye on long-term changes
   Progress Over Time: Pay more attention to long-term trends and changes than you do to short-term ups and downs.

10. Put well-being first:

Prioritize your overall health and well-being as a last resort. If you believe the diet is hurting your health or quality of life, you might want to change it or stop following it altogether.
   Keep in mind that every person's response will be unique; no one solution works for everyone. You can modify the Carnivore Diet to meet the requirements and preferences of your body. You can make wise decisions and get the best results from your diet with regular self-evaluation, self-awareness, and professional medical advice.

Chapter 9: Frequently Asked Questions

Here are some typical queries about the carnivore diet and their responses:

What is the Carnivore Diet, exactly?
A1: The Carnivore Diet is a way of eating that emphasizes avoiding plant-based foods while consuming a lot of animal-based foods. While avoiding fruits, vegetables, grains, and other foods derived from plants, it emphasizes foods like meat, organ meats, and animal fats.

The Carnivore Diet is safe, right?
A2: The Carnivore Diet's safety depends on each person's health status and how well it is planned. Before beginning, seek advice from a medical professional, especially if you have underlying health issues.

What foods are allowed on the carnivore diet?

A3: Meat-based foods like beef, poultry, fish, organ meats, and eggs are acceptable. Dairy products and some animal fats are also acceptable. Fruits and vegetables, which are made of plants, are not included.

Can I get all the nutrients I need from eating only animal products?

A4: Although animal foods offer a variety of nutrients, nutrient deficiencies may develop in the future. Including a variety of animal foods and considering supplements could help with this.

Q5: Can the Carnivore Diet help me lose weight?

A5: Since the Carnivore Diet places a strong emphasis on protein and restricts carbohydrates, many people have reported losing weight while following it. Individual outcomes, however, can vary.

The Carnivore Diet is appropriate for athletes, right?

A6: The Carnivore Diet may be appropriate for athletes due to its higher protein content, which can support muscle growth and maintenance. For intense training, carb needs may need to be taken into account.

If I have a medical condition like diabetes or heart disease, can I still follow the carnivore diet?

A7: Blood sugar and cholesterol levels may be impacted by the carnivore diet. It's essential to work with a healthcare professional to monitor your health markers and make adjustments as necessary if you have these conditions.

A8: Could the Carnivore Diet have any negative effects?

A8: During the transition, some people may experience digestive changes, such as constipation or diarrhea. If not properly managed, nutrient deficiencies and electrolyte imbalances can also happen.

When following the Carnivore Diet, can I still practice intermittent fasting?

A9: Intermittent fasting and the Carnivore Diet are compatible. However, before beginning, speak with a healthcare provider because fasting may impact particular medical conditions.

Q10: Is the Carnivore Diet long-term sustainable?

A10: There is controversy surrounding the Carnivore Diet's long-term viability. Due to the diet's restrictions, some people might find it difficult. Some people might find modified versions that include some plant-based foods to be more sustainable.

Q11: Can I gain muscle mass while following a carnivore diet?

A11: Yes, the Carnivore Diet's high protein content can promote muscle growth. Getting enough calories and exercising properly is crucial for building muscle.

Q12: Can anyone follow a carnivore diet?

A12: Without proper medical supervision, the Carnivore Diet is not advised for those who are pregnant, nursing, have children, or have certain medical conditions.

A registered dietitian or healthcare professional should be consulted before beginning any new dietary approach, including the Carnivore Diet, to ensure that it is in line with your health needs and goals. Keep in mind that individual responses vary.

Addressing Typical Worries And Misunderstandings

To accurately inform people and assist them in making decisions, it is crucial to address common worries and misconceptions about the Carnivore Diet. Here is a thorough explanation of some typical worries and misunderstandings:

1. **A lack of variety in nutrients**

   A lack of dietary variety and nutrient deficiencies could result from excluding plant foods.

   Despite the Carnivore Diet's restrictions on food variety, animal products provide a wide range of nutrients. Nutrient concerns can be reduced by consuming eggs, organ meats, and various animal sources.

2. **Lack of Fiber:**

   Concern: Cutting out plant foods could result in insufficient fiber intake and digestive problems.

   As a result of the low-carb nature of the diet, fiber may not be necessary for everyone. However, adding bone broth and low-carb vegetables may be helpful if you experience digestive problems.

3. **Possibility of Having High Cholesterol:**

   The high intake of saturated fat in the diet raises the risk of heart disease and cholesterol.

There is conflicting evidence regarding the effects of saturated fat on heart health. Concerns can be addressed by keeping an eye on cholesterol levels and working with a healthcare professional.

4. **Lack of certain nutrients**

Concern: Cutting out plant foods could result in vitamin, mineral, and antioxidant deficiencies.

Despite the high nutrient content of animal foods, monitoring nutrient levels and considering supplements can help prevent deficiencies.

5. Energy Shortage:

Concern: The diet's low carbohydrate intake could result in insufficient energy.

Response: After becoming accustomed to the metabolic changes brought on by the diet, many people report sustained energy levels.

6. **Digestive Distress:**

Concern: Changing to a diet high in meat may cause gastrointestinal discomfort.

Response: You can manage digestive problems by gradually introducing new foods, drinking plenty of water, and taking into consideration digestive-friendly foods like bone broth.

7. **Environmental and ethical issues:**

Concern: Ethical and environmental concerns are exacerbated by the production of animals for food.

Choose animal products from sources that are sustainable and think about ethical substitutes, but some people may decide to seek a more balanced diet as a result of these worries.

8. **Insufficient Long-Term Studies**:
Long-term scientific studies on the carnivore diet are scarce.

There haven't been many extensive studies on this particular diet. Short-term studies and anecdotal evidence offer some understanding, but long-term health effects remain poorly understood.

9. **The Carnivore Diet vs. Ketosis:**
Myth: The ketogenic diet and the carnivore diet are interchangeable.

Clarification: While both diets are low in carbohydrates, the Carnivore Diet forbids the consumption of any plant foods, whereas the Ketogenic Diet emphasizes the consumption of high-fat, low-carb foods derived from a variety of sources.

10. Ignoring the Health Benefits of Plants:
Myth: By avoiding plant-based foods, you will forfeit any potential health advantages.

Clarification: Even though plants have distinct health advantages, some supporters contend that animal foods can deliver crucial nutrients and help with particular health objectives.

Sustainable for All, 11.

Myth: The Carnivore Diet is healthy and appropriate for everyone.

Clarification: Reactions vary from person to person, and the restrictive nature of the diet may not be appropriate or sustainable for some groups, such as women who are pregnant or those who have particular medical conditions.

12. **Excessive Focus on Protein:**
Myth: The diet places a lot of emphasis on consuming protein.

Clarification: Although protein is the main focus, consuming enough fat is also very important. In general, the diet encourages the consumption of fatty meat cuts.

To address worries and misconceptions, both sides of the debate must be considered. Before making dietary decisions like the Carnivore Diet, people should carefully weigh the available information, take into account their unique health requirements, and consult with healthcare professionals.

Managing Social Interactions And Going Out To Eat
While managing social situations and eating out while on the Carnivore Diet can present particular difficulties, you can get through these situations successfully with some preparation and communication. How to handle social gatherings and eating out are as follows:

Inform Others of Your Dietary Preferences:

Provide Advance Notice: If at all possible, provide advance notice of your dietary restrictions to hosts or restaurant staff.

1 Simply State Your Case: You can state that you eat primarily meat and other animal products in your diet for health-related reasons.

2. Pack Your Lunch:

Prepare Meals: If you're going to a gathering, think about making dishes that are suitable for carnivores to share with others.

Bring Snacks: In case there aren't many options when eating out, bring portable carnivore snacks like beef jerky or canned sardines.

3. Select Carnivore-Friendly Dining Options:
   Look up restaurants that specialize in serving meat-based dishes, such as steakhouses or barbecue joints.

Call the restaurant ahead of time to discuss your dietary requirements and find out if they can meet your preferences.

4. Personalized Orders:
   Request Modifications: Do not be afraid to request changes to the dishes that are already served. Request a steak, for instance, without any seasonings or sauces.

5. Highlight Meat Selections:
   Prioritize protein: Look for meat-based dishes like steaks, grilled chicken, or seafood on the menu.

6. Be Willing to Change Sides:
   Limited Plant Options: Concentrate on the primary protein source and be flexible with sides because many side dishes may not be compatible with your diet.
   Keep Hydrated:

Drink water, unsweetened tea, or black coffee as your beverage of choice.

8. Justify Your Decisions:
   Educate: If someone asks you about your diet, you can give a succinct justification for choosing the Carnivore Diet.

9. Mingle and Have Fun:
   Change Your Perspective: Put more emphasis on enjoying others' company during the meal rather than making it all about the food.

10. Dealing with Curiosity
    Be patient; loved ones may be enquiring or worried. Provide information and politely respond to their inquiries without forcing your opinions on them.

11. Eating Before or Following:
    Pre-Eating: If you're unsure of the options, think about having a small meal before the event to make sure you won't be starving.

12. Avoiding Peer Pressure
    Remain Confident: Don't feel compelled to stray from your diet; instead, stick to it with confidence.

13. Getting Around Buffets:
    Put Protein First: Pick foods high in protein, such as meat and seafood. Steer clear of foods and sauces that are high in carbohydrates.

14. Offer to Cook

Offer to host events so you can serve food that complies with your dietary restrictions.

Always keep in mind that eating out and social gatherings are about more than just food. While maintaining your diet is crucial, making friends and having fun should also be top priorities. You can maintain your goals while participating in social activities and spending quality time with friends and family by being flexible and well-prepared.

Combining Physical Activity And The Carnivore Diet

For many people, combining the Carnivore Diet with exercise can produce favorable results, supporting general health, fitness objectives, and performance. Here's how to combine the Carnivore Diet and exercise successfully:

1. Getting Enough Protein:

Support Muscle Growth: The Carnivore Diet's focus on foods high in protein can help support muscle growth and repair, making it a good choice for active people.

2. Timing of Proteins:
Pre- and post-workout nutrition: To maximize muscle protein synthesis and recovery, eat protein-rich meals before and after workouts.

3. Water intake:

Maintain Proper Hydration: Both general health and athletic performance depend on proper hydration. Throughout the day, especially during and after exercise, drink water.

4. Electrolyte equilibrium:

Replace electrolytes after intense exercise because it can cause electrolyte loss. Think about consuming foods high in minerals, such as organ meats, or taking electrolyte supplements.

5. Energy Requirements

Caloric Intake: When calculating your caloric requirements for the Carnivore Diet, take into account your energy expenditure from physical activity.

6. Considerations for carbohydrates:

Give your body time to adjust to using fats and proteins as energy sources if you're switching to the Carnivore Diet and are used to eating more carbohydrates.

Cyclical Approach: Some people adopt a cyclical strategy, reintroducing modest amounts of carbohydrates to fuel their workouts. Plant foods with low carbs may be included.

7. Fats for Long-Lasting Energy

Include fatty meat cuts in your diet for long-lasting energy during workouts.

8. Track Recovery

Pay attention to your body: For effective muscle repair and complete recovery, a sufficient protein intake and recovery time are essential. Keep track of how your body reacts to exercise.

9. **Nutritional Density**

Micronutrients: Animal products are high in nutrients and offer the necessary vitamins and minerals for healing and good health.

10. **Added Information**

Omega-3s: Because of their anti-inflammatory properties, omega-3 supplements (like fish oil) may be useful.

11. **Personal Variation**

Monitor how your body reacts to the diet and exercise, in your own words. While some people might discover they have more energy, others might require some time to adjust.

12. **Speak with experts**

Healthcare Provider: If you have a specific medical condition, talk to a registered dietitian or healthcare provider to make sure your dietary and exercise choices are appropriate for your requirements.

13. **Set realistic objectives:**

Performance Objectives: Recognize that during the initial adaptation phase of the diet, your athletic performance may be impacted. Set attainable objectives and monitor development over time.

14. **Experiment and make adjustments**

Trial and error: It might take some time to find the best diet and exercise combination that suits your needs. Be willing to experiment and modify your methods.

For many people, combining the Carnivore Diet with exercise can be beneficial. To support your fitness goals and general well-being, it's critical to give proper nutrition, hydration, and recovery a top priority. As with any dietary or lifestyle change, speaking with a healthcare professional can help you make decisions based on your unique needs and objectives for your health.

Chapter 10: Success Stories and Testimonials

Before starting the Carnivore Diet, I experienced frequent digestive problems and energy slumps. Out of curiosity, I decided to try it, and the results were astounding. My digestion significantly improved within a few weeks; there was no more bloating or discomfort. The sustained energy I experienced all day surprised me the most. The dreaded mid-afternoon slump was no longer a part of my life. I was able to focus better at work and take pleasure in my hobbies thanks to my renewed energy. For me, the diet's simplicity was a game-changer, and I'm appreciative of the positive effects it's had on my general well-being.

Please be aware that every person's experiences are unique, so it's important to think about talking to a doctor before making any significant dietary changes.

People who have tried the Carnivore Diet often highlight a variety of experiences, improvements, and challenges in their success stories and testimonials. These accounts offer anecdotal evidence, but they can also shed light on how the diet has affected various individuals. Here are a few illustrations:

1. **Energy gains and weight loss:**
   Following a carnivore diet, some people have experienced significant weight loss and an increase in energy. They frequently blame the diet's emphasis on protein and restriction of carbohydrates for this.
   Resolved digestion-related issues:

The Carnivore Diet has been reported to help people with digestive issues like bloating, gas and irritable bowel syndrome (IBS) feel better. Certain plant foods should be avoided for improved gut health.

3. **Improvement of mood and mental acuity:**
   Numerous testimonies mention improved focus, mood stabilization, and increased mental clarity after starting the diet. Some people think this is because there are potentially fewer inflammatory triggers.

4. **Lessened Autoimmune and Inflammatory Symptoms:**
   Some sufferers of autoimmune diseases have claimed that the Carnivore Diet has helped them feel better by easing symptoms like joint pain, inflammation, and skin problems.

5. **Improved Sports Performance:**
   Sportspeople and fitness fanatics have discussed how the Car-

nivore Diet has improved their performance and recovery. The increased protein intake promotes the growth and maintenance of muscles.

6. **Reduced Cravings and Simplified Eating:**

People value the diet's simplicity because it does away with the need to organize meals around different food groups. They also claim to have less overall appetite and sugar cravings.

7. **Difficulties and Adjustment Period**:

During the adaptation phase, some people had difficulties with fatigue, gastrointestinal discomfort, and changes in bowel habits. Many people do, however, mention that these problems went away as their bodies adapted to the new eating pattern.

Individual Reactions Differ:

Testimonials stress that everyone reacts differently to the Carnivore Diet. It is crucial to use personalized strategies because what works well for one person might not be appropriate for another.

Although these testimonies offer insights into unique experiences, it's important to keep an open mind and understand that they are only anecdotal accounts. Different people may respond differently to the Carnivore Diet, and what works for one person may not work for another. It is advised to seek the advice of registered dietitians or medical professionals before making significant dietary changes to make sure the diet you choose is in line with your needs and health objectives.

Actual experiences of people following the Carnivore Diet

Individuals who follow the Carnivore Diet report a wide range of real-world experiences. While some people claim significant benefits, others might face difficulties. Following are some themes that people have frequently mentioned in light of their experiences:

Positive Encounters:

Weight Loss: Due to reduced carb intake and increased satiety from protein and fat, many people who follow the Carnivore Diet report successful weight loss.

Improved Energy: Some people report feeling more energized all day long, possibly as a result of stabilizing blood sugar levels and effective fat utilization.

Mental Acuity: Some people claim to have better concentration, mental clarity, and less brain fog.

Digestive Improvement: For people who have digestive problems, the simplicity of the diet and the exclusion of specific plant foods can help relieve symptoms like bloating or gas.

High protein and fat levels in animal foods frequently increase feelings of satiety and decrease cravings.

Reduced Inflammation: Some people with inflammatory conditions claim that their symptoms have lessened, possibly as a result of cutting out possible trigger foods.

Challenges and Things to Think About

Transition Period: Some people go through a period of adjustment during which they may feel exhausted or unwell. Usually, as the body adjusts, this gets better.

Social Situations: It can be difficult to navigate social gatherings, eat out, and respond to inquiries about the diet from friends and family.

Concerns about nutrient diversity may arise if plant foods are eliminated from the diet. To increase their nutrient intake, some people find ways to include organic meats or dairy.

Personalization is necessary: While some people thrive on an all-meat diet, others might need to include plant foods to achieve their healthiest selves. It's critical to be adaptable.

High-protein diets may make it more important to stay properly hydrated and maintain a healthy electrolyte balance.

Addressing these issues while adhering to the diet can be difficult and may call for additional factors to be taken into account.

Lack of Research: The Carnivore Diet's sustainability and

potential health risks are questioned by scant scientific research on its long-term effects.

Individual Variability: Diet responses can vary greatly from person to person, and what is successful for one person may not be successful for another.

It's critical to remember that every person's experiences are unique and influenced by a variety of variables, such as genetics, health, level of activity, and personal preferences. It is advised to speak with medical professionals or registered dietitians before making any significant dietary changes, such as switching to the Carnivore Diet, to make sure that they will support your individual needs and health objectives.

Diverse Viewpoints And Results

The complexity of individual responses to dietary changes is reflected in the varied perspectives and results regarding the Carnivore Diet. The experiences of individuals can be extremely positive or difficult, and these various viewpoints provide a well-rounded understanding of the diet's potential effects. Here is a thorough justification of various viewpoints and results:

1. Positive viewpoints

Health Improvements: Some people report noticeably better digestion, energy levels, weight management, and mental clarity. They credit the removal of plant foods that could be problematic for these beneficial changes.

Athletic Performance: Due to the high protein content and nutrient density of animal foods, athletes and fitness enthusiasts may experience improved endurance, muscle recovery, and strength on the Carnivore Diet.

Autoimmune Conditions: Some sufferers of autoimmune conditions have reported success in reducing pain, inflammation, and other symptoms. These advantages may result from plant foods being free of allergens or irritation-causing substances.

Simpleness: Due to the Carnivore Diet's simplicity and lack of complicated meal planning or calorie counting, many people find it to be simple to follow. This may result in less anxiety when making food decisions.

2. Difficult Experiences:

Adaptation Period: For some people, the Carnivore Diet's initial transition can be difficult and cause symptoms like fatigue, gastrointestinal discomfort, and changes in bowel habits. The length and intensity of this adaptation phase vary.

Social and Emotional Impact: Due to the restrictions of the diet, navigating social situations and eating out can be difficult. Emotional health can be impacted by feelings of loneliness or the need to defend dietary decisions.

Leaving out plant foods raises questions about possible nutrient deficiencies. To ensure they get a variety of important nutrients, people may need to carefully plan their diets.

Sustainability Over Time: Some people believe that the restrictive nature of the diet is not sustainable over time. This may make it difficult to stick to the diet and even cause you to resume your old eating habits.

3. Personal Reactions:

Biochemical Individuality: Every person responds to the Carnivore Diet in a different way depending on their genetics, metabolism, health, and lifestyle choices.

Diverse Objectives: People follow the Carnivore Diet for a variety of reasons, including weight loss, improved health, performance enhancement, or experimentation. Goals affect how people view success.

Genetic Predisposition: An individual's response to the diet may be influenced by how well they tolerate particular dietary components, which may be determined by genetic factors.

4. A Well-Rounded Viewpoint

Flexibility and moderation: Some people follow a modified carnivore diet that occasionally includes plant foods. This strategy aims to strike a balance between the potential advantages of animal foods and the variety of nutrients in plant foods.

Personal Experimentation: Many people see the Carnivore Diet as an experiment, and they're willing to change their strategy in response to how their bodies react and their health objectives.

The Carnivore Diet, in conclusion, elicits a diverse range of viewpoints and results. While some people notice significant improvements in their health and general well-being, others might struggle and find it hard to stick to the diet's restrictions. Genetics, medical conditions, goals, and personal preferences all influence how each person responds. It is advised to speak with medical professionals or registered dietitians before starting the Carnivore Diet or making any significant dietary changes to make sure that the choices suit each person's needs and objectives.

Chapter 11: Moving Beyond the Carnivore Diet

Phase Of Maintenance And Long-Term Plans

Maintaining your health, well-being, and eating habits after leaving the Carnivore Diet depends on the maintenance phase and long-term strategies. The maintenance phase can be approached and long-term plans established as follows:

1. Progressive Integration
   proceed gradually Continue reintroducing foods, just as you did during the transition. Your body can now adapt to a wider variety of foods thanks to this.

2. Nutrient Variety: Adopt a healthy, well-balanced diet that is

rich in a variety of foods, such as fruits, vegetables, lean proteins, whole grains, and healthy fats, as well as dairy if tolerated.

3. Portion Management
   Take Note of Your Body: Pay attention to your hunger and fullness cues and practice portion control. Do not overindulge or severely restrict yourself.

4. Observe Energy Levels
   Observe Well-Being: To make sure you're taking care of your body's needs, keep an eye on your energy levels, mood, digestion, and general health.

5. Performing Regular Exercise
   Continue to be physically active regularly to support your metabolism, muscle health, and general well-being.

6. Achieve Goals
   Adapt Based on Goals: Whether it's weight maintenance, muscle gain, or increased endurance, adjust your dietary choices to coincide with your ongoing health goals.

7. Intentional Eating
   Savor Meals: Engage fully in your meals to practice mindful eating. This can encourage satisfaction and help prevent overeating.

8. Fluids and fiber
   Prioritize hydration: To aid in digestion and gut health, drink plenty of water and eat foods high in fiber.

9. Offer Rewards

Treats Occasionally: Enjoy occasional indulgences guilt-free. To keep a positive relationship with food, balance is essential.

10. Regular Evaluations

Check-Ins: Regularly assess how your body is handling a balanced diet. Over time, changes might be required.

11. Advice for healthcare professionals

Consult Frequently: Arrange routine examinations with medical professionals or registered dietitians to evaluate your health markers and get specialized advice.

12. Adaptability and Flexibility

Stay Flexible: Be willing to change your diet as your health, objectives, and lifestyle change.

13. Sustainable Mentality

Lifelong Approach: Take a lifelong approach to your eating habits, focusing on sustainable decisions that advance your general health.

14. Variety and Pleasure

Food enjoyment: Take pleasure in a variety of foods and flavors. Long-term satisfaction is more likely to come from a varied diet.

15. Mind-Body Relationship

Continue to pay attention to your body's cues to indicate hunger, fullness, and satisfaction.

16. Emotional and Mental Health

Address Well-Being: Give your mental and emotional health a top priority. Long-term success may be facilitated by a healthy, mood-enhancing diet.

Finding a balanced and sustainable eating pattern that supports your health, lifestyle, and goals is the focus of the maintenance phase and long-term strategies. To make sure you're making decisions that advance your general well-being, it's important to be adaptable, self-aware, and willing to seek professional advice when necessary.

Incorporating Learned Lessons Into General Lifestyle Decisions

A crucial step toward a well-rounded and long-lasting approach to health and well-being is incorporating the lessons you've learned from your experience with the Carnivore Diet into your general lifestyle choices. Here is how to apply these lessons to your daily life:

1. Consider Your Experience
Consider the positives and negatives of your experience with the carnivore diet, as well as any difficulties you may have had.

2. Recognize Sustainable Practices
Positive Habits: List the Carnivore Diet behaviors that improve your health and general well-being. These might include consuming more protein, eating slowly, or consuming less sugar.

3. Accept the Diversity of Diets
Embrace Variety Include a variety of foods from all food groups that are nutrient-dense in your diet. Give whole foods and minimally processed foods a top priority.

4. Continue to Eat Mindfully:
Develop mindful eating habits by continuing to pay attention to hunger and fullness signals, savor flavors, and eat with intention.

5. Macronutrients in Balance:
Balanced Approach: Aim for a macronutrient (carbohydrate, protein, and fat) intake that is in balance with your goals and meets your requirements for energy.

6. Keep Hydrated:
Water consumption: Make sure you get enough water throughout the day. Drinking enough water is essential for good health.

7. Adaptability and Flexibility:
Openness to Change: Be flexible enough to adjust to your body's shifting requirements and shifting health objectives. Be flexible with your dietary preferences.

8. Talk about mental and emotional well-being:
Mental and Emotional Well-Being: Take into account how your dietary decisions will affect your emotions and mental health. Give foods that promote mental health top priority.

9. Performing Regular Exercise:

Active Lifestyle: Keep up your regular, enjoyable physical activity. The foundation of a healthy lifestyle is exercise.

10. Consistent Health Checkups:
Health Evaluations: To keep track of important health indicators, monitor your well-being, and get professional advice, schedule regular checkups.
Sustainable Mentality:

Long-Term Approach: Rather than focusing on quick fixes, concentrate on creating enduring habits that improve your health and well-being over the long term.

12. Customized Strategy:

Recognize that your dietary and lifestyle decisions are particular to you. It's possible that what works best for someone else won't be best for you.

13. Ongoing Education:
Stay Up to Date: Keep an open mind and a curious mind when learning about nutrition, wellness, and health. Keep up with reliable information sources.

14. Balance and Self-Care:
Holistic Approach: Put self-care first, control your stress, and strike a balance between your diet, exercise, sleep, and downtime.

15. Honor Achievements:
Celebrate your victories and landmarks achieved on the

road to better health and well-being by acknowledging your accomplishments.

You can develop a holistic view of health by incorporating the Carnivore Diet's lessons into your overall lifestyle decisions. You can develop a long-lasting way of life that supports your well-being by fusing the positive aspects of your Carnivore Diet experience with a variety and balanced approach to eating, physical activity, and self-care.

Chapter 12: Conclusion

Overview of a carnivore diet

The Carnivore Diet is a dietary strategy that places a focus on eating foods with an animal source while avoiding foods with a plant source.

Primary Ideas:

Meat, fish, poultry, eggs, and animal fats make up the majority of it.

Vegetables, fruits, grains, and legumes are among the plant foods that are excluded.

The objective is to satisfy all dietary requirements with animal products.

Historical Background and Prominence:

The diet has a long history and is different in indigenous cultures.

It rose to popularity in the modern era as a result of experimentation and health problems.

Distribution of Macronutrients:

The diet prioritizes consuming protein and fat and is low in carbohydrates.

Density of Nutrients:

Animal products are nutrient-dense and a good source of protein, vitamins, and minerals.

Potential advantages

improvements in body composition and weight loss.

Regulation of blood sugar and insulin sensitivity.

inflammation may occasionally be lessened.

the treatment of some autoimmune diseases.

meal planning made it easier.

Potential negatives

a narrow range of nutrients due to the exclusion of plant foods.

Initial adjustment period with possible exhaustion and digestive problems.

Environmental and ethical issues with animal agriculture.

Risks to one's health and a lack of extensive research.

Integration and Transition:

Reintroduce plant foods gradually to return to a balanced diet. Emphasize portion control, hydration, and nutrient diversity. Personalization and sustainability

The Carnivore Diet is successful for some people over the long term, but it may need to be modified or plant foods should be added back in.

Individual responses vary; for tailored advice, speak with healthcare professionals.

Approach to a Balanced Lifestyle:

Apply the knowledge you've gained from the carnivore diet to your general way of living.

Accept mindful eating, a balanced diet, consistent exercise, and holistic well-being.

Keep in mind that every person's experience with the Carnivore Diet will be different. It is advised to speak with medical professionals or registered dietitians before making any significant dietary changes to make sure your decisions are in line with your needs and health goals.

Encouragement For Making Wise Food Choices

It's imperative to make knowledgeable dietary choices, including those about the Carnivore Diet if you want to improve your general health and well-being. Here is some inspiration to help you through this procedure:

1. Put your health first:

Keep in mind that your most valuable asset is your health. Making informed decisions and investing the time to educate yourself will improve your well-being.

2. Look for Information from Reliable Sources

Collect data from reliable sources like academic studies, licensed doctors, and registered dietitians. Be wary of fad diets and anecdotal claims.

3. Take into account unique factors:

Everybody has a different body. When choosing a diet, take into account your lifestyle, genetics, medical history, and health goals.

4. Moderation and Balance:

The key is balance. Aim for a balanced intake of nutrients from a variety of food sources while researching various dietary strategies.

5. Try New Things Carefully:

If you decide to try the Carnivore Diet or any other new eating regimen, do so mindfully and pay attention to how your body reacts.

Pay Attention to Your Body:

Signals about what works and what doesn't come from your body. Be mindful of your physical, mental, and emotional well-being.

7. Advice from a professional:

Before making major dietary changes, speak with medical professionals like doctors and registered dietitians. Depending on your health situation, they can provide you with tailored advice.

8. Flexibility and Adaptation:
Be willing to modify your dietary preferences in light of fresh information and your personal experiences. Flexibility enables a sustainable strategy.

9. Pay Attention to Long-Term Health
Instead of thinking about quick fixes, consider the long-term advantages of your dietary decisions. Put your health and well-being before obtaining immediate results.

10. Honor Small Successes:
Making wise dietary choices requires effort. Achieving better health and self-awareness is something to be proud of.

Always keep in mind that choosing a diet that is right for you and in line with your values and health goals is the key to making an informed choice. It involves growing, changing, and putting your well-being first above all else.

A Focus On Uniqueness And Bio-individual Reactions
It is essential to emphasize individuality and bio-individual responses when thinking about the Carnivore Diet or any dietary strategy. Here are some reasons why uniqueness is important and how it relates to the Carnivore Diet:

1. Distinct Physiology
Every individual has a different physiological makeup, which

includes genetics, metabolism, and state of health. One person's solution might not be suitable for another.

2. Biological Individuality

Bio-individuality acknowledges that no one diet works for everyone. Due to individual needs, what is advantageous for one person might not be for another.

3. Diet-Body Relationships

Your body's reaction to a particular diet is influenced by a variety of variables, including your genetics, gut health, hormonal balance, and previous dietary habits.

4. Individuality and the Carnivore Diet:

The Carnivore Diet can elicit a wide range of reactions. While some people may thrive on an all-meat diet, enjoying better health and energy, others may experience difficulties or discover that it is unsustainable.

5. Elements That Affect Reactions

Your body's response to the diet can be influenced by variables like age, gender, activity level, health conditions, and personal preferences.

6. Observation and experimentation

Approach any diet you try, including the Carnivore Diet, as an experiment. Make adjustments based on your own experiences after observing how your body responds.

8. Flexibility and Adaptation

Be willing to change your diet based on your bio-individual

reactions. The secret to discovering what suits you best is flexibility.

9. Sustainability over time
   Your dietary decisions will be sustainable and contribute to your long-term health and well-being if you take into account your uniqueness.

10. Keep Comparisons Away
   Do not evaluate your accomplishments or experiences in comparison to others. Your particular journey matters the most because everyone's journey is different.

11. Promote Self-Care: In the end, any diet, including the carnivore diet, should support your overall health and well-being. Put choices that help you achieve your personal health goals first.

Keep in mind that while testimonials and shared experiences can offer useful information, your diet should be based on your bio-individual responses. Pay attention to your body's signals and make decisions that suit your particular needs, preferences, and situation.